Explaining AuDHD

Dr Khurram Sadiq is a Consultant Neurodevelopmental Psychiatrist and leads the ADHD services at Oxleas NHS Foundation Trust and the South East London Integrated Care System. Specializing in autism and ADHD, he is an expert in neurodivergent care pathways and a global speaker on the topic, having delivered six TEDx talks and a speech at United Nations Vienna about neurodiversity. His niche areas are neurodevelopmental conditions, gaming, social media and compassionate leadership.

Explaining AuDHD

Dr Khurram Sadiq

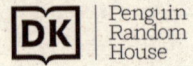

First published in the United Kingdom in 2025 by

August Books, an imprint of
Canelo Digital Publishing Limited,
20 Vauxhall Bridge Road,
London SW1V 2SA
United Kingdom

A Penguin Random House Company
The authorised representative in the EEA is Dorling Kindersley Verlag GmbH.
Arnulfstr. 124, 80636 Munich, Germany

Copyright © Dr Khurram Sadiq 2025

The moral right of Dr Khurram Sadiq to be identified as the creator of this work has been asserted in accordance with the Copyright, Designs and Patents Act, 1988.
All rights reserved. No part of this publication may be reproduced or transmitted in any form or by any means, electronic or mechanical, including photocopy, recording, or any information storage and retrieval system, without permission in writing from the publisher.
No part of this book may be used or reproduced in any manner for the purpose of training artificial intelligence technologies or systems. In accordance with Article 4(3) of the DSM Directive 2019/790, Canelo expressly reserves this work from the text and data mining exception.

A CIP catalogue record for this book is available from the British Library.

Print ISBN 978 1 80436 948 7
Ebook ISBN 978 1 83598 212 9

Printed and bound in Great Britain by Clays Ltd, Elcograf S.p.A.

Look for more great books at
www.augustbooks.co | www.dk.com

Table of Contents

Chapter 1: Introducing the Basics of Autism and AuDHD	1
Chapter 2: Autism	16
Chapter 3: ADHD	38
Chapter 4: When Autism and ADHD Overlap	61
Chapter 5: The Rise of AuDHD	102
Chapter 6: Is AuDHD a Separate Diagnosis?	155
Chapter 7: Towards a Better Understanding of AuDHD	178
Acknowledgements	205
Further Reading	208
Bibliography	211

Chapter 1: Introducing the Basics of Autism and AuDHD

The Revelation

On 4 February 2022, I lost my father. It was the worst time of my life and, simultaneously, it provided the biggest evolution of my life as well. As I was grieving, his life played out like a movie in my head. It's strange that you start to find the missing puzzles of a person's existence once they are gone.

As I reflected on my father's life, I realised that beneath his meticulousness, honesty and principled nature, there was a side of him that was impulsive, reckless and constantly battling with insomnia. These traits, which I had observed throughout my life, suddenly made sense when I began to understand the complexities of Autism and ADHD. It was during my work – conducting assessments that look for both Autism and ADHD – that I saw how different these conditions can appear when they intersect, compared to when they are diagnosed separately. This understanding brought a painful but necessary clarity about my father's struggles.

For years, he had lived with these challenges unknowingly, without proper support or understanding. It became evident to me that his difficulties were not just personal quirks but manifestations of a neurodevelopmental condition that had gone unrecognised. This realisation highlighted a broader issue that affects many people. Individuals who remain undiagnosed or are misdiagnosed often find it incredibly challenging to navigate their lives. They may face difficulties in self-advocating or being accepted, even within communities that are supposed to be inclusive of neurodiversity.

This lack of understanding can be profoundly isolating. People like my father might not be fully accepted by other neurodiverse individuals, who may not recognise the atypical presentation of their conditions, nor by neurotypical people, who might misinterpret their behaviours entirely.

My own journey through grief allowed me to see these patterns more clearly and motivated me to use my father's story as a catalyst for change. I created a framework aimed at helping others who might be in similar situations, giving them the tools and knowledge to find their own path and to navigate a world that often fails to recognise their unique needs. Through this framework I hope to provide guidance and support to those who, like my father, have struggled in silence, helping them to find acceptance and a clearer sense of direction.

This idea eventually became something more – and I felt it was important enough to share with a wider audience. I decided to apply to TEDx, one of the most respected platforms for public speakers. After being rejected ten times, I finally got accepted by a local TEDx event in Las Vegas, a city known for being both misunderstood and full of life. It felt like the perfect place to share my message. The process wasn't easy: it took me six months of grieving and reflecting, working with two TEDx coaches, and going through fifteen drafts to finally shape my talk. On 22 October 2022, which was also my mother's birthday, I had the privilege of presenting my talk: 'When Order and Anarchy Live Together: Autism and ADHD Living in Symbiosis' at TEDxUNLV (University of Nevada, Las Vegas).

Neurodevelopmental Training in the UK

In the UK, formal training in neurodevelopmental conditions is often not a standard part of medical training programmes. This means that many professionals who work in this area have not received comprehensive or specialised training. As a result, those who choose to work in the field of neurodevelopmental conditions often do so out of a personal passion or deep interest in these complex and often misunderstood conditions.

Many professionals in this field are neurodivergent themselves, which means they have first-hand experience of the challenges and strengths that come with Autism, ADHD or other neurodevelopmental conditions. Their personal experience drive them to better understand and support others who face similar challenges; it is also a powerful motivator and provides them with a unique perspective that is invaluable in their work.

Others are drawn to the field because of a fascination with the intricate and sometimes enigmatic nature of neurodevelopmental conditions. They may be intrigued by how these conditions affect the brain, behaviour and overall development, and seek to unravel the mysteries that surround them. These individuals often view the study of neurodevelopmental conditions as a way to contribute to a deeper understanding of human diversity and to improve the lives of those who are affected.

In both cases, whether motivated by personal experience or intellectual curiosity, these professionals often go above and beyond in their efforts to understand and support individuals with neurodevelopmental conditions. Their dedication to the field helps to fill the gaps left by the lack of formal training, and their work is crucial in advancing the understanding and treatment of these conditions in the UK.

Training and Early Years

When I was doing my first-year training in 2005, my consultant asked me to review a patient with Asperger's syndrome. I solemnly asked, 'What is Asperger's?' And he replied, 'Autism.' So then I asked, 'Is he disabled?' My consultant stopped what he was doing, looked up at me and said, 'Go and read about it before assessing the patient.' As I started reading, I got drawn into this world of unknown bounds that were enticing, intriguing and mystifying. The patient turned out to be an astrophysicist. It was the first of many thousands of brilliant conversations with some amazingly talented neurodivergent people.

Five years later, I was asked to lead and pioneer the first adult ADHD and Autism Spectrum Condition (ASC) service in Manchester, where my love affair with neurodevelopmental conditions started. At the time, we were not able to diagnose both conditions simultaneously – it was either/or. It was not until the *Diagnostic and Statistical Manual of Mental Disorders, Fifth Edition* was released in 2013 that both conditions could be diagnosed simultaneously, though off-licence: a specialist could still treat underlying ADHD in an Autism patient, calling it hyperactivity.

What is AuDHD?

AuDHD stands for Autism and ADHD. It is not a formal nomenclature, but how the neurodiversity community and support groups like to refer to those with co-occurring Autism and ADHD. The origin of the terminology is not yet clear, so no one knows who coined it. It helps to define AuDHD's nuances and presentation, as well as distinguishing how it differs from ADHD and Autism individually and acknowledging the ever-increasing co-occurrence of these two conditions.

A 2022 article published in *Frontiers in Psychiatry* discussed that the co-occurrence of Autism Spectrum Condition (ASC) and Attention Deficit Hyperactivity Disorder (ADHD) is estimated to be between 50–70 per cent. This significant overlap underscores the complex relationship between the two conditions, which often presents challenges for diagnosis and clinical management (Hours, Recasens, & Baleyte, 2022).

Living with AuDHD

I vividly remember a woman in her mid-fifties who sought an ADHD assessment with me. As we began, she confided in me that she had delayed this assessment for nearly three decades. She struggled to reconcile how she could be exceptionally organised in certain aspects of her life, yet deeply disorganised in others. Throughout the years, various people had suggested that she might be on the Autism spectrum or have ADHD, but the uncertainty of her condition left her unable to pursue a diagnosis, leading her to postpone the assessment for so long. Her story is a poignant reminder of the challenges many face in understanding and identifying their own neurodiverse experiences.

The patient had endured a long history of misdiagnoses and ineffective treatments, with none of the labels she had been given fully capturing the complexity of her experience. She shared that over the years she had consulted with no fewer than ten psychiatrists, yet she remained an unsolved mystery. As she recounted her symptoms, I couldn't help but smile. Catching this, she paused and asked me about my reaction. I replied with a gentle assurance: 'It's nothing to worry about, but I believe I may finally be able to offer you the answers you've been searching for over the past thirty years.'

I have frequently encountered individuals diagnosed with either Autism or ADHD, only to discern underlying traits of the other condition within them. These traits, existing on the opposite end of the neurodevelopmental spectrum, often stand out to me in ways that seem to elude the observation of other professionals. It has become increasingly clear to me that the nuanced interplay between Autism and ADHD is sometimes overlooked, resulting in a more complex picture that requires a deeper level of awareness and understanding. My experience has underscored the importance of a comprehensive approach in recognising and addressing these intertwined characteristics.

A particularly striking moment occurred during an ADHD assessment when I inadvertently dropped my laptop charger. My patient's reaction was one of pronounced hypervigilance – far more intense than I had anticipated. Initially, I dismissed it as a reflexive response to the sudden noise. However, when the same level of heightened alertness resurfaced after the charger fell again, producing a loud bang, I began to suspect something deeper at play – specifically, sensory overload.

This suspicion led me to further investigate potential autistic traits in my patient, beyond the scope of ADHD. As I delved deeper, a previously overlooked and undiagnosed layer of Autism began to emerge. Signs such as sensory sensitivities, aversion to eye contact, and discomfort in social settings became evident. These autistic features had quietly existed beneath the surface of her ADHD symptoms and been a source of confusion for the patient, as her ADHD diagnosis alone did not fully account for her experiences. It was only through the lens of AuDHD that her unique neuropsychological profile finally made sense, providing her with a more complete understanding of the challenges she faced.

These experiences shows the importance of looking beyond the surface and recognising the intricate overlap between Autism and ADHD, as well as highlighting the need for comprehensive evaluations to better understand and support individuals with these co-occurring conditions.

In my professional experience, some of the most captivating learnings occur when, quite unexpectedly, I uncover the presence of an additional, contrasting, neurodevelopmental condition – such as Autism while assessing for ADHD, or vice versa. These moments of serendipitous exploration not only broaden my understanding of the intricate interplay between these conditions but also underscore the complexity and individuality of each person's neurodevelopmental profile. It is in these instances that the nuanced, multifaceted nature of AuDHD truly comes to light, revealing the delicate balance and interconnection between Autism and ADHD.

The Neurodiversity Paradigm

Recent research has revealed that neurodevelopmental conditions have an evolutionary basis. This discovery supports the Neurodiversity Paradigm: a framework which acknowledges the medical model, but goes beyond it to celebrate and embrace diversity. The Neurodiversity Paradigm recognises the genetic biodiversity and variations among humans, highlighting the unique strengths and perspectives these differences bring.

While the medical model focuses on identifying and describing the deficits associated with neurodevelopmental conditions, often framing them as disorders, the Neurodiversity Paradigm offers a more inclusive and empowering perspective.

It invites us to transcend the conventional view of neurodevelopmental conditions as mere limitations or challenges. Instead, it encourages us to recognise the inherent strengths, unique perspectives and untapped potential that accompany these conditions. This paradigm shift moves us away from the traditional approach of simply managing or mitigating conditions. It calls us to celebrate the rich diversity of human capabilities and the remarkable resilience that individuals with neurodevelopmental conditions often demonstrate.

This broader perspective is foundational to the neurodiversity movement, which actively works to dismantle the stigma surrounding neurodivergent individuals. The movement advocates for a societal shift in perception, urging us to view these conditions not as deficits, but as natural variations in human cognition and behaviour. It challenges the status quo by promoting acceptance, as well as encouraging society to embrace both the strengths and the challenges that come with neurodiversity. In doing so, it fosters an environment where differences are not just acknowledged, but valued, ultimately paving the way for a more inclusive and understanding world.

The Neurodiversity Movement

Jim Sinclair's 1993 piece 'Don't Mourn for Us' stands as a cornerstone in the Autism movement and has significantly contributed to the broader neurodiversity movement. Originally presented at a conference aimed at parents of autistic children, Sinclair's article challenged the prevailing narrative of Autism as a tragedy. Instead of mourning the diagnosis, Sinclair urged parents to embrace and support their autistic children for who they are. The message was clear: Autism is not something to be grieved over, but rather an integral aspect of a person's identity that should be understood, respected and celebrated.

Sinclair's work played a crucial role in advocating for the recognition of neurodiversity – not as a disorder to be cured, but as a natural variation in human experience. By encouraging the acceptance of Autism as a fundamental part of a person's identity, Sinclair's message helped to shift societal perspectives, laying the groundwork for a movement that sees neurodevelopmental differences as sources of strength and diversity rather than deficiencies.

The term 'neurodiverse' or 'neurodivergent' was coined by an autistic sociologist, Judy Singer, in 1998 and became pivotal for the neurodiversity movement. She introduced the concept of neurodiversity to foster a new perspective on neurological differences, viewing them as natural variations within human diversity. Her pioneering work reframed the discourse surrounding conditions like Autism and ADHD, highlighting them in a more positive and inclusive light.

She challenged the medical model, which focuses on deficits and deficiencies. She argued that these conditions are part of the natural diversity of the human brain and advocated for a strengths-based approach that recognises the unique contributions of neurodivergent individuals.

Her ideas resonated deeply with the social model of disability, which asserts that disability results from societal barriers rather than individual impairments. Singer emphasised the imperative for societal transformations to accommodate neurodivergent individuals, focusing on acceptance and support rather than attempts to 'cure' or 'fix' them. The evolutionary perspective on Autism and ADHD reaffirms the Neurodiversity Paradigm ideology.

Evolutionary Perspectives

From an evolutionary standpoint, Autism and ADHD are thought to be ancient neurodevelopmental conditions that have been present since the very origins of humanity. These traits likely served as crucial skill sets that equipped early humans with the tools necessary for survival, adaptation and progress. For instance, the intense focus and attention to detail often seen in Autism may have been invaluable for tasks such as tracking animals or crafting tools, while the high energy and exploratory behaviour associated with ADHD could have driven the curiosity and adaptability needed to navigate and conquer new environments.

As human societies evolved and environmental conditions changed, genetic mutations naturally occurred, leading to variations in how these traits were expressed. In certain tribes or populations, based on their geographical landscapes, the traits associated with Autism and ADHD may have either been advantageous or less so, depending on the demands of their environment. For example, in a hunter-gatherer society, the hyperactivity and quick response times associated with ADHD might have been beneficial for hunting or evading predators. Conversely, in more settled agricultural communities, where routine and repetitive tasks were the norm, these same traits might have become less aligned with the societal demands, leading to what we now see as a mismatch between these genetic predispositions and the modern environment.

This evolutionary mismatch hypothesis suggests that the genetics underlying Autism and ADHD, once highly adaptive, now sometimes conflict with contemporary societal expectations, which are vastly different from those of our ancestors. As a result, what were once essential traits for survival and innovation can now be perceived as challenges or disorders, reflecting a discord between our ancient genetic toolkit and the demands of modern life.

This evolutionary perspective has given rise to another intriguing theory, known as the 'Hunter-Farmer Hypothesis'. This hypothesis explores how the transition from a hunter-gatherer lifestyle to an agrarian society, and eventually to our complex modern societal structures, has contributed to a mismatch between our inherited traits and the current environment.

As we've moved further into modern times, with the development of complex societal structures, industrialisation, and now a predominantly sedentary lifestyle, this mismatch has only deepened. The highly structured, routine-oriented environments of schools and workplaces often do not accommodate the neurodivergent traits that were once crucial for survival. This has led to an increase in the recognition of conditions like ADHD and Autism – not necessarily because these traits are more prevalent, but because they stand out more starkly in an environment that is less aligned with the diverse ways human brains function.

This hypothesis also sheds light on why these conditions might be misunderstood or stigmatised in modern society. The lack of a contemporary environment that appreciates or makes use of the unique strengths associated with ADHD and Autism, combined with societal expectations that favour certain types of behaviour and cognitive functioning, contributes to a gap in understanding. Therefore, many individuals find themselves struggling to adapt to environments that do not cater to their inherent strengths, leading to a perceived increase in these conditions, and a corresponding lack of appropriate support and skill sets to help them thrive.

The Hunter-Farmer Hypothesis, therefore, offers a compelling explanation for the rise in diagnoses of ADHD and Autism, as well as for the challenges in understanding and accommodating these conditions within the context of modern societal and environmental structures. It invites us to reconsider how we design our environments and calibrate societal expectations to better embrace the full spectrum of human neurodiversity.

Evolution of Innovation

Imagine a world where a growing number of individuals boldly embrace and openly share their neurodiversity, becoming catalysts for a profound shift in societal attitudes. These pioneers wear their neurodivergent identities with pride, helping to pave the way for a broader acceptance and celebration of the rich tapestry of human cognition. Their courage and openness serve as a beacon, illuminating the unique strengths and perspectives that neurodiversity brings to our collective experience.

However, even as this transformative movement gains momentum, there are certain groups who misunderstand the essence of neurodiversity. To them it is seen less as a call for genuine understanding and more as a claim to entitlement. This misinterpretation risks overshadowing the true value of neurodiversity, which lies in fostering a deep appreciation for the diverse ways in which people think, learn and interact with the world. The challenge, then, is not just to promote the visibility of neurodivergent individuals, but also to ensure that this visibility is accompanied by a sincere commitment to understanding and valuing their contributions.

In this evolving landscape, it is crucial to foster a culture that not only acknowledges neurodiversity but also deeply understands and respects the unique contributions of neurodiverse individuals. By doing so, we can ensure that the potential of neurodiversity is fully realised for the betterment of society.

In recent years the tech industry has witnessed a significant and encouraging trend: a growing number of companies are actively championing neurodiversity, recognising the invaluable strengths that neurodiverse individuals bring to the workplace. These forward-thinking organisations understand that embracing neurodiversity is not just about inclusivity, but also about tapping into a wellspring of unique perspectives and specialised skills that can drive innovation and enhance productivity. For instance, companies like Microsoft and SAP have implemented neurodiversity hiring programmes, acknowledging that the analytical precision and problem-solving abilities often found in individuals with Autism, for example, can be game changers in fields like software development and data analysis.

These companies are reaping the benefits of fostering an environment where diverse cognitive styles are not only accepted, but also celebrated. By creating inclusive spaces where neurodiverse employees can thrive, they are boosting their bottom lines as well as setting new standards for what a truly innovative workplace looks like.

However, it is disheartening to observe that many companies still lag in this regard. Despite the clear advantages, they remain entrenched in outdated practices, failing to recognise the potential of neurodiverse talent. Instead of embracing these differences, they often scapegoat neurodiverse individuals when challenges arise, overlooking their unique contributions and neglecting their specific needs. For example, in some workplaces employees with ADHD might be unfairly criticised for their difficulty with conventional time management, rather than being supported with tailored tools and strategies that play to their strengths, such as creativity and hyperfocus.

This reluctance to acknowledge and support neurodiversity not only deprives these companies of the innovation and creativity that neurodiverse employees can offer, but also perpetuates a culture of exclusion. As a result, they miss out on the opportunity to build a dynamic, forward-looking workforce that reflects the true diversity of human potential. The challenge for the future lies in encouraging more companies to step out of the shadows and recognise that neurodiversity is not a liability but a powerful asset that, when properly understood and supported, can drive success in ways they have yet to imagine.

To address this disparity and promote a more equitable workplace, many firms are now implementing comprehensive training programmes. These initiatives aim to enhance understanding and appreciation of diversity, creating a fairer and more supportive environment for all employees. By fostering an inclusive culture, these companies champion the rights of neurodiverse individuals while also unlocking a wealth of untapped potential, driving progress and innovation across their industry.

Chapter 2: *Autism*

Autism is a neurodevelopmental condition characterised by impairment in social interactions and communication. For example, people with Autism might not be comfortable with social interactions, finding them deflating and requiring time to recover from them. At a party they might sit in a corner embroiled in their own world, feel uncomfortable or leave the gathering early. They might view small talk as 'pointless' and 'a waste of time'. It's generally only when they get to know someone, and their interests match, that they will indulge in a meaningful conversation. They usually appear to be a closed book and then suddenly explode when emotions overwhelm them. They often struggle to know why they feel the way they feel.

They also often feel indifferent or averse to physical affection. They find it difficult to 'read' the room, such as interpreting emotions and body language, and have to push themselves to observe and analyse. They have a sense of humour that could be characterised as 'different'; they don't find things funny that others do and vice versa; they might be sarcastic but do not understand other people's sarcasm.

They can be literal in their thought process, which makes subtext and metaphor challenging to comprehend. 'I'll be there in five minutes' means the actual five minutes to an autistic person. Once, when I was assessing a young teenager, I asked her to decipher the idiom: 'It's raining cats and dogs.' She replied, 'That's not fair, where are the chipmunks?'

Many individuals with neurodevelopmental conditions often find it challenging to form friendships in the conventional sense. When they do have friends, those friends are usually quite similar to them, often sharing similar neurodevelopmental traits or experiences. People with neurodevelopmental conditions naturally tend to connect with others who understand their unique perspectives and ways of being.

These connections are often formed around shared interests or passions, which serve as common ground for building relationships. Even when such friendships are made, those with neurodevelopmental conditions are rarely the ones to initiate contact or reach out first. More often than not, it is the other person who takes the lead in maintaining the relationship. This dynamic reflects both a comfort in mutual understanding and a preference for deeper, more meaningful connections over social formalities.

Individuals with neurodevelopmental conditions often have discrete interests and love watching the same movies or series repeatedly. They tend to wear similar clothes every day and have a narrow repertoire of food they eat. They like structure and prefer to do things in a certain order. They do not like change or disruption to their routine.

All of these traits can be summed up with the phrase 'the fear of not knowing the unknown' and everything that stems from it. If an autistic individual remains in a consistent environment throughout their life, without transitions, any differences may go unnoticed, as they would be at ease and familiar with all potential outcomes within that setting.

Nomenclature and Definitions

The understanding and terminology of Autism have evolved significantly over the centuries. Since the publication of the *Diagnostic and Statistical Manual of Mental Disorders, Fifth Edition* (DSM-5) in 2013, the medical community has formally referred to it as Autism Spectrum Disorder (ASD). However, within the Neurodiversity Paradigm, the term Autism Spectrum Condition (ASC), or simply Autism, is preferred. This reflects a broader debate over whether to frame Autism as a 'disorder' or a 'condition'.

The neurodiversity movement challenges the notion that neurodevelopmental variations like Autism should be viewed through a lens of deficits. Instead, it emphasises that these conditions should be recognised for their unique strengths and differences. Just as conditions like hypertension or pregnancy are not labelled as diseases or illnesses, but as states of being, many advocate for a similar understanding of Autism. Referring to Autism as a 'disorder' implies a more medicalised perspective, focused on what is lacking or needs to be fixed. Such perspective is increasingly being reconsidered, as society shifts towards a more inclusive understanding of neurological diversity – one that values differences rather than pathologising them.

DSM-5 states that an Autism diagnosis requires persistent deficits in social communication and social interaction across multiple contexts, as manifested by the following: deficits in social-emotional reciprocity, in non-verbal communicative behaviours used for social interaction, and in developing, maintaining and understanding relationships. It also requires having some repetitive and stereotypical behaviours that entail being happy in one's own comfort zone, hence the repetition and having soothing feelings due to the stereotypical movements.

History of Autism

The history of Autism Spectrum Condition (ASC) is a rich tapestry reflecting the evolution of medical understanding, diagnostic frameworks and societal attitudes. The term 'Autism' was coined by Swiss psychiatrist Eugen Bleuler in 1911. He used it to describe a withdrawal from reality, observed as a symptom of schizophrenia, which marked the initial recognition of behaviours later associated with Autism.

In the 1940s, significant strides were made by Leo Kanner and Hans Asperger, who are often credited as pioneers in Autism research. In 1943 Kanner identified a distinct group of children displaying behaviours, such as profound social detachment and a preference for routine, which he termed 'early infantile Autism'. This groundbreaking work uncovered unique patterns in social interaction and communication that laid the foundation for understanding Autism as a separate condition. Concurrently, in 1944, Hans Asperger observed children who, despite autistic traits, demonstrated normal intellectual and linguistic abilities. His findings, later termed 'Asperger's Syndrome', expanded the understanding of Autism's diverse presentations.

The mid-twentieth century was marked by a mix of progress and growing misconceptions. In the 1950s, Bruno

Bettelheim popularised the 'refrigerator mother' theory which posed that a lack of maternal warmth led to Autism. Although influential at the time, this theory was later discredited. In the 1960s, Bernard Rimland's work was pivotal in challenging these outdated notions. His book, *Infantile Autism: The Syndrome and Its Implications for a Neural Theory of Behaviour*, emphasised biological underpinnings, catalysing a paradigm shift towards recognising Autism as a neurodevelopmental condition.

During the 1970s, research increasingly focused on genetic and neurological aspects, moving away from purely psychological explanations. This period marked the beginning of a deeper investigation into the complex interplay of factors contributing to Autism, laying the groundwork for contemporary scientific enquiry.

The 1980s and 1990s brought significant changes in diagnostic criteria to enable clinicians to make better diagnoses. Autism was officially recognised as a distinct disorder in the 1980 DSM-III and classified under Pervasive Developmental Disorders (PDD). This classification underscored the need for specific diagnostic criteria, which were broadened in subsequent DSM editions. The 1987 edition of DSM mentioned Pervasive Developmental Disorder – Not Otherwise Specified (PDD-NOS) and included atypical cases which didn't completely fit all of the established diagnostic criteria.

In 1994, DSM-IV introduced a more nuanced classification, with five distinct conditions under the PDD umbrella, including Autistic Disorder, Asperger's Disorder, Childhood Disintegrative Disorder and Pervasive Developmental Disorder – not otherwise specified. Rett syndrome does not come under the ASD diagnostic criteria anymore because, unlike Autism

Spectrum Condition (ASC), it usually starts with a period of normal development after which children begin to lose skills they had previously acquired. Children with Rett syndrome often experience significant difficulties with motor skills, which is not as common in ASD. Rett syndrome also has specific features, such as irregular breathing patterns, seizures and a unique hand-wringing motion – none of which are typical signs of ASD.

The twenty-first century marked a shift towards a spectrum-based understanding of Autism. Increased media attention and advocacy led to greater public awareness, fostering a more inclusive perspective. In 2013, DSM-5 unified previously separate diagnoses into Autism Spectrum Disorder (ASD), reflecting the new recognition of the condition's diverse manifestations. ASD was characterised by impairments in social communication and restricted, repetitive behaviours, with severity levels introduced to describe the required support.

In 2018, the International Classification of Diseases (ICD-11) adopted a similar spectrum approach, listing ASD as a single condition with varying degrees of severity and impairment. This alignment in diagnostic frameworks represented a global consensus on the spectrum nature of Autism.

Throughout its history ASD has transitioned from being misunderstood and stigmatised to being recognised as a complex neurodevelopmental condition with a strong genetic basis. Modern perspectives emphasise a dimensional approach, appreciating the wide variability in how Autism manifests across individuals. This evolution in understanding underscores the importance of continued research, advocacy and support for those on the Autism spectrum.

Autism is a Learning Disability

For many years Autism was mistakenly thought to be a type of learning disability. While it is true that some individuals with learning disabilities may also have Autism, Autism itself is not a learning disability. People with Autism may face challenges with learning, such as difficulties with reading, writing or understanding complex information. However, these challenges stem from differences in how their brains process and interpret the world rather than from a specific learning disability. Autism primarily affects how people perceive and interact with others and the world around them, and each person with Autism has their own unique strengths and difficulties.

Autism is Caused by Emotionally Distant Mothers

There is a common misconception, widely portrayed in popular culture, that psychologist and therapists tend to blame parents for most mental health problems.

The 'refrigerator mother' theory is a now discredited idea suggesting that Autism in children was caused by emotionally cold and distant mothers. This theory emerged in the 1950s and 1960s, heavily influenced by psychoanalytic perspectives prevalent at the time. Pioneered by Leo Kanner and later championed by Bruno Bettelheim, the theory posited that mothers who were not warm or nurturing enough were the primary cause of Autism in their children.

Kanner's initial research observed a perceived lack of warmth among the parents of autistic children, which he proposed might have contributed to the development of

Autism. Bettelheim expanded on this notion, suggesting that the emotional detachment of mothers could be likened to the coldness of a refrigerator, thereby coining the term 'refrigerator mother'. He went further and controversially compared the emotional environments in these homes to the harsh conditions of concentration camps, highlighting the perceived detrimental impact on children.

By the late 1970s the 'refrigerator mother' theory faced substantial criticism and was largely discredited. Emerging research began to emphasise the genetic and neurological foundations of Autism, thereby challenging and undermining the simplistic cause-and-effect relationship that the theory suggested. The 'refrigerator mother' theory had severe implications for mothers, leading to feelings of guilt, shame and isolation. Many mothers internalised the blame, which adversely affected their mental health and societal perceptions.

Autism Only Affects Males

Significant research on Autism has predominantly focused on white males. For a long time, it was believed that the condition manifested almost exclusively in males, which meant that studies into females with Autism were very limited.

Evidence-based research has traditionally estimated the male-to-female ratio for Autism Spectrum Condition (ASC) to be around 4:1, indicating that Autism is diagnosed approximately four times more often in males than in females.

However, more recent studies suggest that this ratio may not accurately reflect the true prevalence of Autism in females, which often manifests differently than in males, leading to underdiagnosis or misdiagnosis. Females with Autism may display less obvious signs or develop stronger social coping skills, making their condition less recognisable under the traditional diagnostic criteria, which were largely developed based on male characteristics.

Taking these differences into account, some research suggests that the actual male-to-female ratio might be closer to 3:1 or even 2:1. This implies that Autism in females may be more common than previously believed but often underrepresented in diagnostic statistics due to its unique presentation and the challenges in recognising it.

Autism is Caused by the MMR Vaccine

In 1998 Andrew Wakefield, a British physician, along with twelve colleagues, published a groundbreaking article in the esteemed medical journal *The Lancet*. The article suggested a potential link between the MMR vaccine – designed to protect against measles, mumps and rubella – and the onset of Autism in some children. This assertion, despite being later debunked due to faulty data interpretations, had a profound impact on vaccination rates across both the United Kingdom and the United States, as more parents refused to have their children inoculated.

The controversy resurfaced in 2016, with the release of the documentary *Vaxxed*, which alleged that the Centers for Disease Control (CDC) were concealing evidence of a connection between the MMR vaccine and Autism. Independent scientists and specialists have since refuted these claims, reaffirming that there is no evidence to support any link between the MMR vaccine and Autism. Nonetheless, the conspiracy theory has stubbornly persisted, particularly within the United States.

In 2004 investigative journalist Brian Deer published a series of revealing articles that exposed numerous conflicts of interest involving Andrew Wakefield, the lead author of the original study. Deer uncovered that the study had been funded by a lawyer named Barr, with promises of additional compensation for Wakefield if the study was accepted. Furthermore, Deer revealed that Wakefield had applied for a patent for his own vaccine, using his personal address and contact information. In the wake of these revelations, ten of the twelve co-authors of the initial study retracted their support, collectively acknowledging that there was no causal link between the MMR vaccine and Autism.

This series of events underscores the significant influence of flawed research and the enduring power of misinformation, even in the face of overwhelming scientific evidence.

Two pivotal studies played a crucial role in dispelling the myth that the MMR vaccine is linked to Autism.

The Finnish Study (2000)

> The Finnish study conducted by researchers from the Hospital for Children and Adolescents in Helsinki followed 1.8 million individuals over 14 years, starting from the introduction of the MMR vaccination programme in 1982 (Pediatric Infectious Disease Journal, 2000;19:1127-34). By the end of 1996, nearly three million doses of the vaccine had been administered. During this period, 173 potentially serious adverse events were recorded as possibly

linked to the vaccine, with febrile seizures being the most common occurrence.

Importantly, no cases of inflammatory bowel disease or autism were identified during the study. The researchers concluded that if there were any association between the MMR vaccine and these conditions, the prospective design of the study would have revealed at least some cases, thereby reinforcing the safety of the MMR vaccine.

The Danish Cohort Study (2002)

In the early twentieth century, a team led by Kreesten Meldgaard Madsen embarked on an extensive research project in Denmark. This large-scale study encompassed all children born in the country between 1991 and 1998, totalling over 537,000 participants. The researchers meticulously compared the incidence of Autism between vaccinated and unvaccinated children. Their comprehensive analysis revealed no increased risk of Autism in those who received the MMR vaccine compared to those who did not. This study provided robust and compelling evidence against the hypothesis that the MMR vaccine causes Autism.

These studies, through their thorough methodologies and large sample sizes, have been instrumental in reaffirming public confidence in the safety of the MMR vaccine, demonstrating unequivocally that it does not contribute to the development of Autism.

Andrew Wakefield's study, published in *The Lancet* in 1998, had a notably small sample size involving only twelve children. The limited scope of this sample significantly undermined the study's validity. Moreover, the research was marred by substantial methodological flaws, including selection bias and a lack of rigorous controls. These issues were critical factors in the study's subsequent retraction and the widespread debunking of its findings by the scientific community.

Despite its eventual retraction, the study caused a significant decline in vaccination rates in both the United Kingdom and the United States. In the UK, vaccination rates dropped from over 90 per cent to around 80 per cent, leading to outbreaks of measles, mumps and rubella. These diseases, once under control, resurged, resulting in serious health complications and even deaths.

In response to the crisis, the scientific and medical communities conducted extensive research to reaffirm the safety of the MMR vaccine. Health organisations intensified efforts to educate the public on the importance of vaccines, emphasising the lack of credible evidence linking them to Autism.

However, the misinformation from Wakefield's study fuelled a persistent vaccine hesitancy movement, which has remained entrenched, and also gave rise to various conspiracy theories about vaccine safety and government cover-ups.

Autism Is a New Concept

Autism is a heritable neurodevelopmental condition. People are born with it and it is passed on from one generation to another. Autism is under a high degree of genetic control and suggests the involvement of multiple genetic loci.

There is a new branch of psychiatry called evolutionary psychiatry which has established that Autism was once a skill set, a survival toolkit that helped humankind survive the perilous environments that endangered their existence.

Individuals with high-functioning Autism may have had survival advantages due to their exceptional memory, spatial skills and expertise in specific areas, particularly in traditional societies where solitary foraging could improve survival chances.

The persistence of Autism, despite its potential disadvantages for individuals, may be explained by group selection theory, which suggests that traits beneficial to the group, even if detrimental to individuals, can persist through evolutionary history. The resurgence of this theory highlights the potential historical advantages of having individuals with high-functioning Autism within ancestral hunter-gatherer tribes. Today, the value of high-functioning individuals in various roles is increasingly recognised and appreciated.

People with Autism Lack Empathy

The general perception is that people with Autism lack empathy, which is something that involves understanding another's mental state and responding appropriately. Most people with Autism have very fixed facial expressions, struggle with eye contact and possess a monotone voice. They are unable to communicate feelings, hence the apparent lack of empathy.

One can divide empathy into components of cognitive empathy (understanding another person's perspective) and affective empathy (emotional responses to others' mental states). Both are crucial for social functioning. Individuals with ASD often exhibit atypical empathic responses, which can hinder communication and social interactions.

The connection between Autism and empathy is complicated and varied. Research has shown that autistic people can have very different experiences with empathy. Some might feel others' emotions very strongly (hyper-empathy), while others might have a harder time understanding others' perspectives (cognitive empathy). Also, different studies have used different definitions of empathy, which has led to mixed results.

Hyper-empathy in some autistic people can result from past trauma, making them very sensitive to others' feelings and therefore making social interactions difficult. Therapy can help to reduce these intense feelings by addressing the underlying trauma.

The theory of mind, which is the ability to understand what others are thinking, is often seen as impaired in autistic individuals. However, it is important to understand that the ability to grasp others' thoughts and feelings is not completely absent in people with Autism. Many on the Autism spectrum can develop these skills to some extent, especially with guidance and time. While it may not come naturally to them, some learn to use different approaches to understand what others might be thinking or feeling.

Recent studies have also revealed that theory of mind itself exists on a spectrum and people, whether on the Autism spectrum or not, show different levels of ability to understand others' perspectives. This more nuanced view challenges the misconception that individuals with Autism lack this ability altogether, instead emphasising the wide range of experiences and capabilities within the autistic community.

However, some experts argue that both autistic and non-autistic people struggle to understand each other: a concept known as the 'double empathy problem'.

Double empathy is a concept that suggests that misunderstandings in communication and empathy do not only happen because people with Autism struggle to understand non-autistic people, but also because non-autistic people often have difficulty understanding those with Autism. Essentially, it's a two-way street where both sides can struggle to see things from the other's perspective.

It was thought that people with Autism had a lack of empathy or difficulty understanding social cues. However, the idea of double empathy challenges this by suggesting that the problem arises because of a mismatch in communication styles and perspectives. People with Autism may understand each other quite well and communicate effectively among themselves. Similarly, non-autistic people also tend to understand each other easily. The breakdown happens when these two groups try to interact, leading to misunderstandings on both sides.

The double empathy concept highlights the importance of recognising that everyone has unique ways of seeing the world and that social challenges between autistic and non-autistic people are not one-sided. It's about bridging the gap in understanding between different perspectives and fostering better communication by appreciating these differences.

Many autistic people find it hard to identify and describe their own emotions, which is something called alexithymia, from the Greek words *a*, meaning lack or without, *lexis*, meaning word, and *thymos* meaning emotions or feelings. Roughly translated, alexithymia means 'a lack of words for emotion'.

Overall, our understanding of empathy in Autism is improving, as we now recognise the wide range of experiences and the need for more nuanced approaches in research and social interactions. This helps to better support and understand autistic individuals.

Autism Can Be Cured

I met a woman with AuDHD who shared her experience of going through an assessment. She took great care in choosing professionals who truly understood neurodiversity, and everything seemed to be going smoothly. However, at the end the assessor made a comment: 'Don't worry, we can cure you.' Upon hearing this, she immediately ended the interview and left. She was deeply upset, knowing that Autism is not a disorder, but a condition people are born with, and is not something that needs to be cured like a disease. This is a typical misperception both among professionals and the lay public.

Autism is a neurodevelopmental condition with a genetic basis involving multiple genes, for which there is no pharmacological treatment. Increasingly, people are advocating for it to be recognised as a condition rather than a disorder.

Among children, Autism support is about incorporating their skill set, with behavioural techniques and parental training. In adults, it's about developing insight about the condition and finding answers to questions. There are some incredible books out there, such as *Pretending to be Normal*, which is the biography of an autistic girl and her journey that helped so many people understand what Autism is.

Assessment and Diagnosis

When diagnosing Autism, I generally use the DSM criteria rather than the International Classification of Diseases (ICD), because I find that the former offers a more in-depth and nuanced approach to understanding neurodevelopmental conditions. Diagnosing Autism is not a simple process, as it involves looking at the individual's experiences from all angles to gain a full picture. This means carefully examining behaviours and traits from childhood, and understanding how they have evolved and manifest in adulthood. Only by taking this comprehensive, 360-degree view can we accurately connect the dots between early signs and current behaviours, leading to a more accurate diagnosis.

For children and adults – though more relevant for children – the assessment typically includes a social play observation and an Autism Diagnostic Observation Schedule (ADOS) assessment. The latter is a widely used assessment tool designed to help professionals understand if someone might be on the Autism spectrum. It involves a series of structured activities and conversations that allow the assessor to observe a person's social, communication and behavioural skills in real time.

During the ADOS assessment, the individual is guided through various tasks and interactions, such as playing with toys, having a conversation or completing puzzles, depending on their age and language ability. The activities are designed to create opportunities to see how the person communicates, how they use eye contact and gestures, how they understand social cues, and how they respond to different situations.

By watching how the person behaves in these scenarios, the assessor can gather important information about their social and communication strengths and challenges. The ADOS is considered one of the most reliable methods for assisting in diagnosing Autism as it provides a structured way to observe behaviours that are key indicators of Autism, rather than relying solely on interviews or questionnaires.

Overall, ADOS helps to create a clearer picture of an individual's social and communication abilities, which can guide a more accurate diagnosis and provide insights for support and intervention.

This is followed by gathering a developmental history, either through clinical interviews, or tools like the ADI-R, DISCO or the *Royal College of Psychiatrists Diagnostic Interview Guide for the assessment of Adults with Autism Spectrum Disorder(ASD)*.

The Autism Diagnostic Interview-Revised (ADI-R) is a comprehensive tool used by professionals to help diagnose Autism in both children and adults. It involves a structured interview conducted with a parent or caregiver who knows the person well. This covers several key areas and is designed to gather detailed information about the individual's developmental history and behaviours related to social interaction, communication and repetitive or restricted behaviours.

Questions about early development help identify any signs of Autism that may have appeared in childhood, such as delays in speech or difficulties in social engagement. The interview also explores how the person communicates, both verbally and non-verbally, as well as their ability to form relationships and understand social cues. Additionally, it looks into any repetitive movements, routines or specific interests that are often characteristic of Autism.

This in-depth interview process allows the clinician to gain a thorough understanding of the individual's behaviour patterns and developmental history. The insights gained from the ADI-R help to determine if the person meets the criteria for an Autism diagnosis and to identify the type of support or interventions they may need. Therefore, ADI-R is considered a valuable tool in providing a clear and accurate diagnosis, guiding both treatment planning and support strategies.

The Diagnostic Interview for Social and Communication Disorders (DISCO) is an in-depth assessment tool used to help diagnose Autism and other developmental conditions. Developed by Lorna Wing and her colleagues at the National Autistic Society in the UK, DISCO is designed to capture a comprehensive view of an individual's behaviours, social interactions, communication skills and developmental history.

Unlike some other diagnostic tools that may focus narrowly on certain behaviours or symptoms, DISCO takes a holistic approach. It involves a structured yet flexible interview with a parent, caregiver or someone who knows the person well, as well as direct observations.

One of the key strengths of DISCO is its ability to identify the subtleties and nuances of Autism spectrum conditions across the lifespan. It does not only help in diagnosing Autism, but also in understanding the individual's needs and how best to support them. The DISCO's framework is grounded in the concept that Autism is a spectrum, where individuals can exhibit a wide variety of traits and behaviours, allowing for a more tailored and person-centred approach to assessment.

The questions in DISCO are extensive and cover a wide range of areas, including early development, communication abilities, social interactions, play, interests and adaptive behaviours. This breadth allows clinicians to gain a deep understanding of the person's strengths, challenges and unique profile. After these steps, a comprehensive report is prepared.

Both psychologists and psychiatrists can conduct these assessments, but they must be trained in these specific tools. Before starting the formal assessments, I usually gather information from parents, siblings and close relatives to ensure a holistic perspective.

Management of Autism

Managing Autism involves a comprehensive and personalised approach that addresses the unique needs and strengths of each individual. Since Autism affects people differently, the management plan must be flexible, combining a range of therapies, supports and strategies to promote development, improve social and communication skills, and enhance daily living.

Early support is essential, as programmes that focus on building communication, and social and motor skills can make a significant difference in a child's development. Educational settings that provide individualised learning plans tailored to a child's way of learning can help them thrive. Behavioural support, such as positive behaviour strategies and emotional coping techniques, can also play a crucial role in managing challenges and building essential life skills.

Speech and occupational therapies are vital in helping individuals to improve communication and daily living skills. Social skills training teaches how to interact with others, understand social cues and form meaningful relationships. Additionally, family education and support are crucial, as they empower relatives to provide the best possible care and guidance for their loved ones.

Medical care is also an important aspect, particularly for managing co-occurring conditions like anxiety or ADHD. Sensory integration therapy helps individuals to manage sensitivities to sounds, lights or textures, while assistive technology can provide alternative ways to communicate and support independence. Effective management of Autism requires a person-centred approach, regular monitoring, and adaptation of strategies to ensure they remain relevant and supportive as the individual grows and their needs evolve. This holistic approach aims to create an environment that encourages growth, independence and a high quality of life.

Recent Developments in Autism

Recent developments in Autism research have led to major advancements in understanding and potential treatments. Scientists have discovered how certain genetics for Autism affect the brain, providing insights that could lead to more targeted treatments. New ways to deliver drugs to the brain are also being explored. These include the use of advanced technologies to get genetic material directly into the brain, potentially allowing for treatments that are customised to each person's genetic make-up and therefore will be pivotal in genetic syndromes.

Additionally, early Autism screening has made significant progress. The National Institute of Mental Health (NIMH) has helped to improve early detection and intervention. Early screening tools like the Modified Checklist for Autism in Toddlers (M-CHAT) now allow us to identify Autism as early as twenty-four months. This early detection means we can start helping kids much sooner, which greatly improves their long-term development.

The ASD Pediatric, Early Detection, Engagement and Services (ASD PEDS) Network has played a key role in these efforts, screening over 109,000 children and developing effective methods for early diagnosis and treatment.

Scientists have identified over a hundred genes related to Autism, helping us understand more about its causes. They've found specific changes in the brain linked to these genes, which is a big step towards creating targeted treatments.

Chapter 3: ADHD

ADHD, which stands for Attention Deficit Hyperactivity Disorder, is a neurodevelopmental condition that individuals are born with. The characteristics and symptoms associated with ADHD are present from early development and can impact various aspects of life as the individual grows. The term ADHD may not fully encapsulate the broad range of symptoms and challenges it represents. Many argue that it focuses too narrowly on hyperactivity and inattentiveness, missing other crucial elements of the condition.

Inattention is not unique to ADHD; it is also a feature of several other mental health conditions, such as anxiety, depression and Autism. What sets ADHD apart and determines its diagnosis is the specific pattern and combination of symptoms which include inattention, hyperactivity and impulsivity.

Diagnosing ADHD involves a comprehensive evaluation that includes a detailed history, symptoms assessment, and often input from multiple sources such as parents, teachers and healthcare providers. This thorough approach ensures that the diagnosis accurately reflects the individual's experiences and helps to differentiate ADHD from other conditions with overlapping symptoms.

Features of ADHD

Individuals with ADHD, often referred to as ADHDers, are frequently characterised by their seeming carelessness and inattentiveness. They can be easily distracted by apparently trivial stimuli, such as a bird chirping, a car screeching or someone entering the room. Even their own thoughts can pull their focus away, making it challenging to stay on task. This heightened distractibility stems from the way their brains are wired, making it difficult for them to filter out irrelevant stimuli and maintain attention on a single task.

Procrastination, although not officially part of the diagnostic criteria for ADHD, is a significant and pervasive feature. Those with ADHD often find themselves zoning out during conversations, lessons, meetings and lectures. They might miss crucial pieces of information, leading to repeated requests for clarification on topics that have already been covered. This tendency to lose track of discussions and presentations can create barriers to learning and effective communication, further complicating their daily lives.

This pattern of behaviour is a manifestation of the underlying neurological differences that define ADHD. The condition affects the brain's executive functions, which are crucial for managing time, organising tasks and maintaining focus. As a result, ADHDers often struggle to complete assignments, follow through with plans and meet deadlines, leading to a cycle of frustration and self-doubt. Understanding these challenges is key to providing appropriate support and developing strategies to help them navigate their environment more effectively.

ADHDers often find it challenging to maintain focus on activities such as reading or watching a film. They generally have shelves brimming with unfinished books, and their online streaming platforms reveal a plethora of incomplete series and movies. During a film, they might frequently get up to tend to other tasks, or to grab snacks or drinks, causing any shared viewing experience to stretch much longer than usual as they struggle to stay engaged from start to finish.

A common characteristic of ADHD, seen in both children and adults, is a tendency to daydream or become lost in thought. This can happen at any moment, even during conversations or when they need to focus on a task. Their attention may drift away, making it difficult for them to stay engaged with what is being discussed. As their minds wander, they might suddenly shift to talking about completely unrelated topics, leaving others confused or feeling like they are not being listened to. This habit of mentally drifting off can create challenges in daily life, as it affects their ability to stay present and focused on the moment, whether in school, at work or in personal relationships.

ADHDers often experience a rapid onset of boredom, leading them to frequently switch hobbies and become sidetracked by mundane tasks. This behaviour results in a trail of unfinished projects and activities. As children, this tendency manifests as an inability to complete homework, often leaving it until the last possible moment, either early in the morning or just before the lesson begins. The underlying issue is a lack of stimulation, which drives procrastination and ultimately leads to a crisis and last-minute efforts. On the other hand, ADHDers often excel when working under tight deadlines, as the pressure and potential consequences, whether incentives or criticism, provide the necessary motivation to complete tasks efficiently. This can sometimes lead to periods of hyperfocus.

Administrative tasks can be particularly challenging for individuals with ADHD because they demand skills that do not come easily to them. These chores often require quick and timely responses, careful organisation and meticulous attention to detail to be completed properly – all of which can feel overwhelming. For someone with ADHD, staying focused on paperwork, keeping track of deadlines or sorting through documents can be daunting. The need to manage multiple steps, prioritise effectively and maintain concentration can make these tasks feel exhausting and frustrating, leading to procrastination or incomplete work. As a result, what might seem like simple, routine tasks to others can feel like an uphill battle for someone with ADHD.

The complexity and structured nature of administrative work may often lead to frustration and a sense of being overwhelmed, which then further exacerbates their struggles with maintaining focus and completing tasks efficiently.

ADHDers often struggle with organisation, a challenge that can be vividly illustrated by their personal living spaces. Their rooms are more likely than average to be described as 'bomb sites', with items strewn across the floor in what some humorously call a 'floordrobe'. Clothes, wrappers, dirty dishes, cups, books and toys often pile up in chaotic heaps, reflecting their difficulty in maintaining order.

This disorganisation extends beyond physical spaces. People with ADHD tend to overcommit, agreeing to take on numerous tasks or appointments. They might double-book themselves, arriving either too early or too late for engagements. Despite creating to-do lists and schedules, they frequently find it challenging to follow through, resulting in many unchecked items and rigid calendars that serve more as scaffolds than actual guides.

Forgetfulness is another hallmark of ADHD. It's common for individuals to misplace everyday items like phones, keys or passports – a phenomenon often referred to as the 'ADHD tax'. These items might turn up in unusual places, such as refrigerators or bathrooms, causing panic when they cannot be found. Forgetting to pay bills or return calls is also typical, necessitating constant reminders.

For schoolchildren this forgetfulness might mean leaving important items at home or school, further complicating their daily routines and requiring frequent prompts from parents or teachers. Understanding these organisational challenges is essential for developing strategies that can help to manage and mitigate the impact of ADHD on daily life.

ADHDers often exhibit a high degree of restlessness and an inability to remain still, which becomes particularly noticeable in structured settings such as classrooms or meetings. This restlessness can manifest as leg bouncing, fidgeting with objects in their hands, or a constant need to get up and move around. The physical discomfort associated with sitting still for prolonged periods makes it challenging for them to focus on the task at hand.

Relaxation is another area where individuals with ADHD face significant challenges. They are unable to unwind and relax without doing, or thinking about doing, something else. They often appear hyperactive and constantly on the go, with an energy level that can be both infectious and exhausting for those around them. This perpetual motion is not just a physical trait but extends to their thoughts and speech as well. They may come across as loud or overly chatty, often lacking the internal cues to know when to stop talking. This can lead to disruptive behaviour, as they inadvertently dominate conversations or interrupt others.

Impulsivity is a core characteristic of ADHD that affects various aspects of behaviour. Those with ADHD may struggle with self-control, leading to actions without considering the consequences. For children, this might manifest as impatience in taking turns, darting into the street without caution, or finding it difficult to wait in line. Adults may sometimes exhibit intense road rage, such as when another driver cuts them off; they might resort to using profanities, making rude gestures, tailgating or even stepping out of their vehicle to confront the other driver. This reflects a broader tendency towards impatience and an urgent need for immediate gratification. They often desire things to happen right away, so are willing to pay extra for a parcel to be delivered as quickly as possible or become frustrated when waiting for a meal to arrive. These behaviours highlight a broader difficulty in maintaining boundaries and respecting the social norms that govern patient and deliberate action.

The combination of restlessness, hyperactivity and impulsivity creates a dynamic but challenging environment for individuals with ADHD and those around them. Understanding these traits can help to develop effective strategies to manage symptoms and improve interpersonal interactions.

In simpler terms, ADHD can be thought of as a constant need for stimulation. This condition is largely due to an imbalance in the brain's neurotransmitters, specifically dopamine and norepinephrine. These chemicals play a crucial role in regulating attention, hyperactivity, impulsive behaviour, and emotional dysregulation, which is responsible for the symptoms seen in ADHD.

According to the DSM-5 and the ICD-11, ADHD is classified into three distinct types, each characterised by different sets of symptoms.

1. Predominantly Inattentive Type

People with this type of ADHD primarily struggle with attention and focus. They find it challenging to concentrate on tasks, are easily distracted, and often have difficulties with organisation and forgetfulness. This might mean they frequently lose things, fail to follow through on instructions, or have trouble keeping their work or living spaces tidy.

2. Hyperactive-Impulsive Type

This is characterised by high levels of activity and impulsivity. Individuals may be very fidgety and unable to sit still for long periods, and they often talk excessively. They might interrupt others, make hasty decisions without thinking through the consequences, and act in ways that can be perceived as disruptive in social situations.

3. Combined Type

This includes symptoms of both inattention and hyperactivity-impulsivity. People with this type exhibit a mixture of the symptoms described above, making it the most comprehensive form of ADHD. They struggle with maintaining focus and organisation, while also being highly active and impulsive.

History of ADHD

The concept of ADHD has evolved significantly over the centuries, rooted in the idea that uncontrolled child behaviour could have a medical explanation.

Historically, in Western societies children were valuable economic contributors to their families, especially in agricultural settings where they could help with farming and other labour-intensive tasks from an early age. With industrialisation, children transitioned from being workers to students and by the early twentieth century that economic value was almost completely deferred until adulthood. This shift also influenced family dynamics, with fewer children per family and an increased emphasis on academic achievement and schooling.

Intellectual movements during the Enlightenment and Romantic periods further shaped the understanding of childhood and behaviour. Thinkers like John Locke and Jean-Jacques Rousseau emphasised the developmental process of learning, and the inherent goodness and curiosity of children. This period saw a growing recognition of children's rationality, leading to the idea that behavioural disturbances could be the result of underlying conditions. Clinicians began to view children as susceptible to conditions that could affect their behaviour, emotions and cognition, laying the groundwork for modern concepts like ADHD.

The earliest recorded ideas about what we now call ADHD can be traced back to 1902 when Sir George Still, a British paediatrician, delivered a series of lectures to the

Royal College of Physicians in London. He described a group of children who exhibited impulsive behaviour, had difficulty paying attention and showed a 'defect of moral control' despite being of normal intelligence. Although his ideas did not gain widespread recognition at the time, his work would later be used to demonstrate that ADHD has deep historical roots and a legitimate medical basis, challenging the notion that it is simply a result of modern parenting styles.

In the 1930s and 1940s, research began to suggest that these behavioural issues might be connected to neurological factors. At that time, the condition was commonly referred to as 'minimal brain dysfunction' or 'minimal brain damage', as it was thought to be the result of subtle brain injuries or abnormalities.

By the 1950s and 1960s, the understanding evolved beyond the idea of brain injury, leading to a broader acknowledgment of hyperactivity as a key feature in children. It was during the 1960s that the term 'Hyperkinetic Impulse Condition' was introduced to describe children who were unusually restless and had difficulty maintaining focus. This term was among the first to specifically highlight hyperactivity: a core characteristic of what we now understand as ADHD.

The term Attention Deficit Disorder (ADD) first appeared in the *Diagnostic and Statistical Manual of Mental Conditions* (DSM-III) in 1980. At that time, ADD was classified with or without hyperactivity, highlighting two distinct types of the condition: one focusing on inattention and the other on hyperactivity.

In 1987, the revised edition of the DSM (DSM-III-R) replaced ADD with Attention-Deficit Hyperactivity Disorder (ADHD), recognising that inattention and hyperactivity-impulsivity could coexist in varying degrees within the same condition. This change marked a more nuanced understanding, acknowledging that it could present in multiple ways.

The 1990s saw further refinement with the publication of the DSM-IV, which identified three subtypes of ADHD: Predominantly Inattentive, Predominantly Hyperactive-Impulsive and Combined Type. This classification allowed for a more accurate diagnosis that could cater to the varying presentations of ADHD in different individuals.

With the release of the DSM-5 in 2013, the understanding of ADHD expanded even more. The criteria now included specific guidance for diagnosing ADHD in adults, recognising that it is not confined to childhood but can persist throughout a person's life. This edition also removed the subtypes, instead recognising them as 'presentations' that can change over time.

ADHD was officially included in the World Health Organization's International Classification of Diseases, 11th Revision (ICD-11), which was released in June 2018 and took effect in January 2022. In the ICD-11, ADHD is classified as a neurodevelopmental condition, characterised by patterns of inattention, hyperactivity and impulsivity that affect a person's daily life. This classification aligns closely with other major diagnostic guidelines and ensures that ADHD is recognised globally as a genuine condition, helping guide proper diagnosis, treatment and support.

The concept of ADHD continued to evolve, influenced by various neurological theories and the impact of medical conditions like encephalitis. Epidemics and conditions such as minimal brain damage were linked to behavioural and cognitive impairments in children. This period also saw the introduction of stimulant medications, which significantly impacted the understanding and treatment of hyperactivity and attention disorders.

Myths and misconceptions about ADHD

You Don't Have ADHD

One prevalent misconception is that achieving academic or professional success negates the possibility of having the condition. Many people believe that gaining entry into prestigious institutions, like medical schools or engineering colleges, precludes an ADHD diagnosis. This assumption is misguided and overlooks the complex reality of the condition.

Patients frequently report that general practitioners deny them ADHD assessments on the basis of their professional achievements or employment status. This narrow viewpoint fails to recognise that high intelligence and strong cultural support systems can mask the symptoms of ADHD. For instance, in cultures such as those in Southeast Asia, Africa and East Asia, children often benefit from robust family support, strict parenting and rigorous educational environments. These structures can provide a scaffolding that helps individuals to manage their symptoms, thereby concealing the underlying ADHD.

Similarly, highly structured environments like boarding schools or careers in the military offer frameworks that support individuals with ADHD, making it less apparent. The rigid routines and clear expectations in these settings can help to mitigate some of the challenges associated with the condition, leading to the mistaken belief that it is absent.

It's crucial to understand that ADHD can affect individuals regardless of their achievements or intelligence. The presence of supportive structures doesn't eliminate the condition but can temporarily obscure its features. Recognising this helps in providing appropriate assessments and support for those with ADHD, ensuring they receive the understanding and treatment they need.

ADHD Only Occurs in Males

The previously observed male-to-female ratio in ADHD diagnoses, which ranged from 3:1 to 4:1, has been steadily decreasing. Historically, diagnostic tools and assessment criteria were predominantly based on studies involving white males, leading to a significant underdiagnosis of ADHD in females.

One primary reason for this disparity is that ADHD often manifests differently in females. Women and girls are more likely to exhibit inattentive symptoms rather than the hyperactive and impulsive behaviours commonly seen in males. Additionally, many females with ADHD develop sophisticated masking and mirroring techniques to cope with their symptoms, making it less likely for their condition to be recognised and diagnosed.

Contrary to previous beliefs, ADHD affects males and females almost equally. The growing awareness of this fact has led to an increase in ADHD referrals and diagnoses among females. This surge reflects a broader understanding of the condition and highlights the importance of developing gender-inclusive diagnostic criteria that accurately capture the diverse presentations of ADHD across different populations.

My Child Doesn't Have ADHD

During ADHD assessments for adults, it is common for parents to dismiss the possibility that their child might have had ADHD. This reaction is influenced by several factors.

Firstly, there is a phenomenon where 'eyes can't see what the mind does not know'. Many parents simply lack awareness of ADHD symptoms and its diverse presentations. They are often unfamiliar with the condition's characteristics, leading them to attribute their child's behaviours to laziness or naughtiness, thus perpetuating common stereotypes.

Secondly, some parents may deny the possibility of ADHD due to a fear of blame. Admitting that their child has ADHD could be seen as a reflection on their parenting, so in order to avoid this perceived criticism, they might reject the idea altogether.

Thirdly, in neurodivergent families where ADHD is prevalent, the behaviours associated with the condition may be seen as normal. This normalisation makes it difficult for family members to recognise ADHD symptoms as distinct or problematic. In such environments, the unique challenges posed by ADHD might go unnoticed because they are part of the household's everyday experience.

Lastly, cultural stigma plays a significant role. In certain cultures, there is a strong stigma associated with any form of neurodivergence or mental health issue. This stigma can lead to a refusal to acknowledge ADHD, as admitting to such a diagnosis could be seen as socially unacceptable or damaging to the family's reputation.

Overall, these factors contribute to the reluctance or inability of some parents to recognise and accept ADHD in their children, complicating the assessment and diagnosis process for adults seeking help for their symptoms.

ADHD Only presents in Children

In 2006, when I presented my research on adult ADHD to a Research Ethics Committee, a consultant psychiatrist openly expressed scepticism about my work, suggesting that it lacked validity. At that time the concept of adult ADHD was not widely recognised in the UK, and lacked acknowledgment and guidelines from the National Institute for Health and Care Excellence (NICE). Back then, there was a common belief that ADHD symptoms would fade away as individuals reached adulthood, typically disappearing by the age of eighteen. This view was widespread and reflected a limited understanding of the condition. It wasn't until 2008 that adult ADHD was officially recognised in the UK, and its understanding and acceptance as a lifelong condition have evolved considerably since then.

The persistence of such myths has been largely due to insufficient psychological education across society. Many professionals and laypeople alike adhere to the outdated view that ADHD is exclusively a childhood condition. This has reinforced the erroneous belief that adults cannot have ADHD, thereby hindering proper diagnosis and treatment for those continuing to struggle with the condition into adulthood.

Fortunately, the landscape is changing. With increased awareness and education, more healthcare providers and community members are recognising that ADHD persists beyond childhood. This shift is crucial for providing appropriate support and interventions for adults with

ADHD, ensuring they receive the necessary care to manage their symptoms effectively.

ADHD Is Overdiagnosed

The prevalence of ADHD is estimated to be 6–10 per cent, whereas the prevalence of schizophrenia stands at approximately 1 per cent. Despite the higher prevalence of the former, there are significantly fewer services dedicated to managing ADHD compared to those for schizophrenia. This discrepancy highlights a critical gap in the availability of care and resources for individuals with ADHD.

There is a substantial backlog of generations of adults over thirty awaiting diagnosis. This oversight can be attributed to a historical lack of awareness, insufficient skill sets among healthcare providers, and an inadequate workforce to address the needs of this population.

The COVID-19 pandemic between 2019 and 2022 acted as a catalyst, leading to a dramatic increase in referrals, because it dismantled the existing structures that many individuals with undiagnosed ADHD relied upon, exacerbating their struggles to remain functional. The sudden removal of these support systems often resulted in crises, necessitating referrals to emergency services and intervention. In some regions, referral rates surged to as high as 500 patients per month.

Contrary to the notion that ADHD is overdiagnosed, the reality is that it remains significantly underdiagnosed. The surge in referrals during the pandemic underscores the urgent need for increased services and resources to support individuals with ADHD.

It's Just a TikTok Diagnosis

It deeply disturbs me when a genuine medical condition is trivialised as a 'TikTok diagnosis'. To fully understand this issue, we must consider the evolution of society and how we access information. Each generation has its unique methods of learning and engaging with information through different media. As a member of Generation X, raised in the 1980s, I grew up in an era where learning was sought through physical media. My father nurtured my quest for knowledge by providing me with a set of *Encyclopaedia Britannica*. We relied on newspapers, and magazines like *Reader's Digest*, *Newsweek*, *Times* and *The Economist* to acquire information and satiate our curiosity.

We now live in the age of Generation Alpha, a highly digitalised generation. It is crucial that we embrace this transition and recognise that the media may change, but the need for discernment remains constant and we must critically evaluate the content we encounter online.

With the advent of the internet, followed by social media, the way we access and share information transformed dramatically. Social media platforms and their short-form content, such as Reels, have become prevalent sources of information, both good and bad, and it is our responsibility to differentiate between the two.

Labelling ADHD as a 'TikTok diagnosis' undermines the genuine struggles and experiences of those affected by the condition. It is not the platform but the quality of information and our ability to critically analyse it that matters. ADHD is a legitimate medical condition that deserves serious attention and understanding, regardless of the medium through which people learn about it. We must continue to advocate for proper education, awareness and support for all individuals with ADHD, ensuring that their condition is recognised and treated with the respect it deserves.

Assessment and Diagnosis

Screening and diagnostic tools for ADHD serve different purposes in the identification and evaluation process.

Screening tools are the initial step and are designed to quickly identify individuals who might have symptoms of ADHD. These tools are often simple questionnaires or checklists that assess common symptoms like inattentiveness, impulsivity and hyperactivity. They help to flag individuals – whether children, adolescents or adults – who may need further evaluation, but do not provide a diagnosis on their own.

Diagnostic tools, on the other hand, are more thorough and are used when screening tools indicate the possible presence of ADHD. They involve a detailed assessment conducted by trained professionals, such as psychologists or psychiatrists, to determine if a person meets the specific criteria for ADHD. The diagnostic process includes in-depth interviews, behavioural observations, and sometimes standardised tests to evaluate a person's history, behaviour patterns and the impact of symptoms across different areas of life. While screening tools help identify who might need further assessment, diagnostic tools are essential for making a formal and accurate ADHD diagnosis.

Diagnosing ADHD is a comprehensive and holistic process that varies slightly between children, adolescents and adults but consistently aims to gather a full spectrum of relevant information from multiple sources.

In diagnosing ADHD in children and adolescents, it is crucial to gather comprehensive information from both schools and parents. Teachers can provide important observations of the child's behaviour in the classroom, while parents offer detailed insights into their child's behaviour and development over a longer period of time. Screening tools like the Conners Rating Scales and SNAP-IV are used to assess these behaviours. The former consist of questionnaires filled out by parents and teachers, helping to identify ADHD-related symptoms such as inattention, hyperactivity and impulsivity. Similarly, SNAP-IV is a checklist that evaluates ADHD symptoms based on responses from both parents and teachers, allowing for a broader view of the child's behaviour in different environments.

The Qb Test adds another layer to the assessment by using a computer-based approach to measure a child's attention, impulsivity and activity levels. It provides objective data that can be compared to typical behaviour patterns, helping clinicians see where a child may differ. For a more structured and comprehensive diagnostic evaluation, tools like the Young DIVA-5 are employed. The DIVA-5 involves a detailed interview with both the child and the parents, covering developmental history, symptoms and their impact on daily life. This ensures a thorough understanding of the child's experiences and provides a well-rounded basis for an accurate diagnosis. These tools together help in creating a clearer picture of the child's behaviour, ensuring that the diagnosis is precise and that the right support and interventions can be put in place.

Diagnosing ADHD in adults requires a thorough, well-rounded approach that takes into account a person's entire life history and current daily functioning. This process involves reviewing past school records and any previous assessments, which can reveal early signs of ADHD that may have been overlooked or misunderstood at the time. Equally important is gathering input from those who know the individual well, such as parents, siblings, partners, close friends or colleagues. Their observations provide valuable context for understanding how the individual's behaviour has manifested across different settings and over the years.

Screening tools play a key role in this process. The Adult ADHD Self-Report Scale (ASRS) is a widely used questionnaire that allows individuals to rate how often they experience symptoms commonly associated with ADHD, such as difficulty concentrating, impulsiveness or restlessness. This self-assessment helps to identify patterns that might suggest ADHD. Similarly, the Wender Utah Rating Scale focuses on childhood behaviour and its continuity into adulthood, which is particularly useful for adults who may not have been diagnosed when they were younger. It provides insight into how past behaviours relate to current challenges. The Conners Adult ADHD Rating Scales offer another layer of assessment by gathering information from both the individual and others around them, such as a spouse or close friend, to provide a balanced view of their symptoms.

To build on the findings from these screening tools, a more detailed evaluation is conducted using tools like the DIVA-5 (Diagnostic Interview for ADHD in adults). This structured interview delves deeply into the individual's experiences, covering both childhood and adult life, and looks closely at the presence and impact of ADHD symptoms. The combination of these tools – self-reports, historical records, observations from others and thorough interviews – ensures that the diagnosis is comprehensive, accurate and reflective of the individual's real-life challenges and experiences. This holistic approach is essential for developing an effective, comprehensive and personalised management plan.

Overall, the diagnosis of ADHD is a methodical process that integrates diverse sources of information and utilises specialised tools. Each assessment session is thorough and detailed, often taking up to three hours cumulatively to ensure that all aspects of the individual's behaviour, history and current symptoms are meticulously examined. This extensive process is designed to ensure that the diagnosis is accurate and that any co-occurring conditions are identified and addressed appropriately.

Management of ADHD

Management approaches for ADHD differ between children and adults. For children and adolescents, the focus is initially on behavioural strategies, social-skills training and parental guidance, with medication introduced if needed. In contrast, for adults, medication is often the first line of treatment, with behavioural techniques, cognitive behavioural therapy (CBT) and coaching used as complementary supports to enhance overall effectiveness.

Medications are generally divided into two categories: stimulants and non-stimulants. Stimulant medications such as methylphenidate (e.g. Ritalin, Concerta) and amphetamines (e.g. Adderall, Elvanse) are the most commonly prescribed. They work by increasing the levels of dopamine and norepinephrine in the brain, which helps to improve focus, attention and impulse control. Adderall, which is a combination of two stimulants, is only licensed in the US at the time of writing.

Non-stimulant medications include atomoxetine (Strattera), guanfacine (Intuniv) and clonidine (Kapvay). These medications may be recommended for individuals who do not respond well to stimulants or who experience significant side effects. They work differently, often by affecting other brain pathways, to help regulate attention and behaviour.

There are some unlicenced medication that can be used, like Modafinil.

Behavioural therapies are also an essential part of managing ADHD. Cognitive behavioural therapy (CBT) is particularly effective in helping individuals to develop strategies to manage their symptoms, such as improving organisational skills, reducing procrastination and learning to manage emotional challenges. Other therapeutic approaches focus on building social skills, improving communication and addressing any co-occurring issues like anxiety or depression.

Combining these approaches – medication, behavioural therapy and ADHD coaching – offers a comprehensive and tailored strategy for managing ADHD, supporting both immediate symptom relief and long-term skill development for a more balanced and fulfilling life.

Recent Developments in ADHD

Precision Medicine

Precision medicine represents the future of ADHD management, utilising pharmacogenomics to tailor treatments to individuals' genetic profiles. By conducting DNA testing, clinicians can identify the most effective medications for each patient, as well as recognising specific food products that may exacerbate ADHD symptoms.

This personalised approach ensures that treatments are optimised for efficacy and minimised for adverse effects, providing a more effective and targeted management strategy for individuals with ADHD.

ADHD Coaching

ADHD coaching has gained popularity as a practical intervention that incorporates techniques from various therapies to enhance daily functioning. Coaches work with individuals to develop skills that improve organisation, reduce forgetfulness, and increase patience and focus. This hands-on approach helps clients to implement structured routines and strategies that mitigate common ADHD challenges, leading to more productive and manageable daily lives.

Mindfulness-Based Interventions

Incorporating mindfulness techniques into treatment plans has shown considerable promise in managing ADHD symptoms. Practices such as meditation and mindful breathing help individuals to develop greater self-awareness and emotional regulation. These interventions can significantly reduce symptoms of inattention and hyperactivity, fostering a calmer and more focused mindset.

Digital Therapeutics and Apps

EndeavorRx is a groundbreaking FDA-approved video game-based therapy designed for children aged 8–12 with ADHD. Through engaging and adaptive gameplay, EndeavorRx targets and enhances specific cognitive functions like attention and focus, making therapy both effective and enjoyable.

Mobile Apps

A growing number of mobile apps are being developed to support ADHD management. They offer features such as medication reminders, symptom tracking and cognitive exercises. AI-based apps like Motion assist users in organising their daily schedules, ensuring they stay on track and manage their symptoms more effectively.

Workplace Strategies

Employers are becoming more aware of the needs of employees with ADHD and are implementing supportive workplace strategies. These include flexible schedules, the use of assistive technologies, and other accommodations that enhance productivity and well-being, ensuring that employees with ADHD can thrive in their professional environments.

By embracing these advancements, from precision medicine to digital therapeutics, the management of ADHD is becoming more personalised, effective and supportive, allowing individuals to lead more fulfilling and productive lives.

Chapter 4: When Autism and ADHD Overlap

ADHD	vs	Autism
Inattention	vs	Indifference
Distraction	vs	Sensory Overload
No Filter	vs	Factual Discourse
Hyperfocus	vs	Preoccupations
Social Inappropriateness	vs	Social awkwardness
Over-talkativeness	vs	Talking Passionately
Impulsivity	vs	Acting Out

Whenever I hear professionals say they cannot tell the difference between Autism and ADHD, I feel a surge of frustration. How can they not distinguish between these two very different conditions? Autism and ADHD have no similarities in their diagnostic criteria and yet professionals often struggle to tell them apart. In this chapter, we will explore why this confusion exists and persists. We will look at what people think of when they consider Autism and ADHD, and how the characteristics of these conditions might overlap.

Let us begin by examining the diagnostic criteria to understand the foundational distinctions. Until 2013, it wasn't possible to diagnose someone with both Autism and ADHD at the same time. This makes me wonder how many people with both conditions, often referred to as AuDHD, might have been overlooked. In the world of neurodevelopmental conditions, AuDHD is still not well understood and is often stigmatised. People find it hard to see the connection between Autism and ADHD because AuDHD doesn't always show clear traits of either condition.

The saying that if you've met one person with Autism or ADHD, then you have met just one person with those conditions holds true for AuDHD as well. Each person with AuDHD is unique, and their experiences and behaviours can't be generalised.

My autistic mind often struggles to grasp how people explain certain things, which can lead to confusion. For example, when I talk about the incidence of AuDHD, I tend to say there's a 50–70 per cent co-occurrence of Autism with ADHD. But I've often been puzzled by how studies present these findings differently. Some suggest that among those diagnosed with ADHD, around 15 per cent also have Autism, while others state that among those with Autism, 30–70 per cent have ADHD. It's quite confusing, isn't it?

Autism in ADHD

They say that the brain often finds clarity in moments of boredom or stillness – those are the times when synaptic connections can form most effectively – and recently, I experienced such a moment that illuminated the intricate and often misunderstood relationship between Autism Spectrum Condition (ASC) and Attention Deficit Hyperactivity Disorder (ADHD). This epiphany came to me while I was exploring the serene and untouched northern areas of Pakistan. For the first time in years, I had taken a break from my work — a full two weeks away from the demands of clinical practice and research. My mind, free from its usual preoccupations, began to unravel the complexities surrounding the overlap between Autism and ADHD, and I started to critically evaluate the prevailing statistics that shape our understanding of these conditions.

One of the most frequently cited statistics is that 'among those diagnosed with ADHD, there is a prevalence of 15 per cent for Autism'. At first glance this figure seems to suggest that ADHD is the more dominant diagnosis, with Autism being a secondary consideration — an afterthought, almost. This reading implies that ADHD characteristics are typically more visible or pronounced, while the signs of Autism are less obvious or less likely to be present. However, such a straightforward interpretation fails to capture the complexity and depth of the overlap between these two neurodevelopmental conditions.

Recent research has challenged this conventional understanding by revealing that the true rate of co-occurrence between Autism and ADHD is substantially higher, with estimates ranging between 50 and 70 per cent. This discrepancy raises critical questions about our current diagnostic practices and the subtleties of symptom presentation. Rather than Autism being a secondary or less significant diagnosis in individuals with ADHD, it appears that the two conditions often coexist in a much more intertwined and interdependent manner than previously thought.

This insight suggests that ADHD can frequently overshadow or 'mask' the traits of Autism, leading to underdiagnosis or misdiagnosis of ASD in individuals initially identified with ADHD. The hyperactivity, impulsivity and inattentiveness associated with ADHD can dominate the clinical picture, making it more challenging to discern the social communication difficulties, restricted interests and repetitive behaviours characteristic of Autism. As a result, the autistic traits may remain hidden beneath the surface, unrecognised by both clinicians and caregivers, who are more attuned to the overt symptoms of ADHD.

The implications of this overlap are profound and multifaceted. Understanding the nuanced relationship between Autism and ADHD is not just an academic exercise; it has real-world consequences for diagnosis, treatment and support. For instance, recognising that these conditions frequently coexist can lead to more comprehensive assessments that consider the possibility of dual diagnoses rather than a singular focus on either ADHD or Autism. Such an approach would facilitate more tailored interventions that address the full spectrum of a person's needs, potentially improving outcomes in both clinical and everyday contexts.

Moreover, this high prevalence of co-occurring symptoms underscores the need for a paradigm shift in how we conceptualise and approach these neurodevelopmental conditions. Rather than viewing ADHD and Autism as discrete entities with occasional overlap, it may be more accurate to consider them as existing on a continuum, where the boundaries are fluid and the manifestations deeply interconnected. This perspective calls for a more integrative framework that recognises the shared neurobiological underpinnings, as well as the complex ways in which these conditions can influence and exacerbate one another.

The intricate interplay between Autism and ADHD requires a more nuanced and informed understanding that goes beyond simplistic statistical interpretations. The significant overlap between these conditions invites us to rethink our diagnostic criteria and clinical approaches, moving towards a more holistic view that embraces the complexity of neurodevelopmental diversity. This realisation is not only a call to action for clinicians and researchers, but also a beacon of hope for individuals and families navigating the often-confusing landscape of these overlapping conditions.

This dual recognition allows for the development of more personalised and effective management plans that cater to the complete range of an individual's needs. In essence, my moment of clarity emphasised the critical importance of recognising the high rate of co-occurrence between Autism and ADHD. It highlighted how ADHD can frequently overshadow the features of Autism, complicating the diagnostic process. By embracing this complexity, we can enhance diagnostic precision and offer more comprehensive support to individuals navigating the intertwined characteristics of these neurodevelopmental conditions, ultimately elevating our clinical expertise and approach.

ADHD in Autism

Contrary to the frequently cited prevalence rates of Autism among those diagnosed with ADHD, the presence of ADHD traits in individuals with a primary diagnosis of Autism is reported to range from 30 per cent to 50 per cent. This statistic suggests that when Autism is the initial diagnosis, identifying co-occurring ADHD can be relatively more straightforward. The hallmark characteristics of ADHD – hyperactivity, impulsivity and inattention – are generally more prominent and visible, and stand out against the backdrop of Autism's core features, making them easier to detect in the clinical setting.

When Autism is recognised first, the subsequent identification of ADHD, particularly the hyperactive-impulsive type, tends to be more direct. The behaviours associated with hyperactivity and impulsivity, such as excessive talking, fidgeting and a need to move constantly, are typically overt and distinguishable.

However, the predominantly inattentive presentation of ADHD presents a more subtle and intricate challenge. Inattention, characterised by difficulties sustaining focus, frequent distractions and forgetfulness, can often be overshadowed by the more defining features of Autism, such as social communication challenges, repetitive behaviours and restricted interests. This overlap can lead to underdiagnosis or misdiagnosis, especially if the inattentive symptoms are relatively mild or if the clinician's focus is primarily on the more conspicuous traits of Autism.

A critical phenomenon that complicates the diagnostic process in these cases is 'masking'. Masking involves individuals with neurodevelopmental conditions developing strategies to camouflage their difficulties, often to conform to societal expectations or to avoid drawing attention to themselves. While masking is frequently discussed in the context of autistic individuals concealing their Autism-related behaviours within an ADHD framework, it is equally pertinent when considering how ADHD symptoms can be masked within an Autism diagnosis. The coping strategies developed to manage social interactions, sensory sensitivities or adherence to routines in Autism can inadvertently conceal the symptoms of inattention typically associated with ADHD.

For example, an autistic individual who appears intensely engaged in a special interest might be misinterpreted as demonstrating 'hyperfocus', a trait commonly linked to ADHD. However, this intense engagement may instead reflect an autistic trait of restricted, repetitive behaviour rather than the concentration difficulties of ADHD. Such overlaps can blur the clinical picture, requiring a nuanced and comprehensive evaluation to disentangle the symptoms and identify the true nature of the individual's neurodevelopmental profile.

While identifying ADHD in individuals already diagnosed with Autism is often less diagnostically complex than identifying Autism in those with an initial ADHD diagnosis, both scenarios require meticulous and thoughtful consideration. The key distinction lies in the visibility of the symptoms: ADHD's hyperactive-impulsive traits are more immediately observable and often stand out against Autism's backdrop, whereas Autism's subtler social communication difficulties and sensory sensitivities can be easily overshadowed by ADHD's more overt behavioural symptoms.

This complexity underscores the need for a careful, layered approach in clinical evaluations. Clinicians must be vigilant in recognising how one condition may mask or mimic the other and ensure that assessments are sufficiently detailed to capture the nuanced interplay of symptoms. By doing so, we can move towards a more accurate understanding of the dual presentation of Autism and ADHD – an understanding that is critical for developing more effective and individualised treatment plans.

Understanding the Nuances of AuDHD

To truly grasp the unique presentation of AuDHD, we must first navigate the intricate landscape of each condition's symptoms. Both ASD and ADHD are characterised by their own sets of core features, and understanding these subtleties is crucial to unravelling the complexities that often blur the lines between them. This foundational knowledge is vital for deciphering the overlapping traits that can lead to confusion, misdiagnosis or even a failure to recognise the presence of both conditions in an individual.

The Overlapping Features of Autism and ADHD

Autism and ADHD, while distinct in their core diagnostic criteria, are both classified as neurodevelopmental conditions and often share certain overlapping features that can appear deceptively similar on the surface. This overlap can make it challenging for clinicians, caregivers and even the individuals themselves to differentiate between the two. However, the overlapping features seen in individuals with AuDHD do not stem from a single source but instead represent the interplay of two distinct neurodevelopmental profiles.

Autism is primarily characterised by difficulties with social communication, restricted interests, repetitive behaviours and sensory sensitivities. On the other hand, ADHD is defined by patterns of inattention, hyperactivity and impulsivity. Despite these distinct diagnostic hallmarks, the two conditions can intersect in ways that obscure their boundaries. For instance, both conditions can manifest as difficulties in maintaining focus, challenges in social interactions, or behaviours perceived as impulsive or rigid. It is within these intersections that the complexities of AuDHD emerge, revealing a blend of characteristics that are not easily categorised as purely autistic or purely ADHD-related.

In individuals with AuDHD, these overlapping traits require a careful and nuanced interpretation to understand their origins. For example, what might be viewed as distractibility in ADHD could, in the context of Autism, reflect an inability to filter out extraneous sensory information. Similarly, hyperactivity in ADHD may overlap with the repetitive motor movements or need for sensory input seen in Autism. Therefore, it is essential to consider both the context and the underlying neurobiological differences that contribute to these manifestations.

By exploring the shared and distinct features of Autism and ADHD, it's clear that these traits originate from separate yet intertwined pathways. This conclusion is a vital step in developing more accurate diagnostic criteria and more effective, individualised support strategies for those navigating life with both Autism and ADHD. The complexity of AuDHD lies in its duality – requiring us to look beyond surface-level behaviours and delve deeper into the cognitive, sensory and social dimensions that define each condition and their convergence in the individuals they affect.

1. Inattention vs Indifference

> **Case Study 1:** Sophie is a seven-year-old child who is bright and creative but struggles significantly with maintaining focus in structured settings. In school, she often daydreams, fails to complete assignments and requires frequent prompts to stay on task. At

home, routine activities like getting dressed or doing chores are challenging due to her easily distracted nature. Although she can concentrate intensely on activities she enjoys, her attention quickly fades for less engaging tasks.

Her inattentiveness affects her academic performance and social interactions, where she sometimes misses social cues, though she is still well-liked for her kindness and creativity.

Case Study 2: Liam, an eight-year-old boy, appears indifferent and disengaged from his surroundings, often showing little interest in both social interactions and activities that other children enjoy. At school, he rarely participates in class or interacts with peers during recess, preferring instead to be by himself or engage in repetitive activities like arranging objects or drawing. His teachers have noted his reluctance to make eye contact or respond to his name unless prompted multiple times.

At home, Liam is more comfortable with routine and familiar settings, resisting new experiences and appearing withdrawn during family outings. His lack of curiosity and engagement also affects his academic performance, which is average but could be improved if he showed more interest in lessons.

Initially, his teachers attributed his behaviour to inattention, but upon closer examination it became clear that it was rooted in a lack of interest and indifference, which is indicative of underlying Autism.

Attention

Attention is the mental ability to focus on specific things, ignore distractions and keep our minds on a task. It's a key part of how we understand and respond to everything happening around us.

Imagine you're a parent trying to get your child ready for school in the morning. Your goal is to make sure they have everything they need and leave on time. Here's how attention works, told through a simple example.

Sustained attention is similar to watching over a child as they get dressed, ensuring they stay on track without getting sidetracked or losing focus. It involves consistently guiding them back to the task at hand whenever their mind begins to wander, or they get distracted by something else. The goal is to help them maintain their concentration and complete the activity from start to finish without drifting away to other interests or activities. Just like this, sustained attention requires continuous mental effort to stay engaged with a single task until it is fully completed.

Focused attention is like the concentration required when tying your child's shoelaces. In that moment, your mind is fully centred on this one specific task, carefully ensuring that each step is done correctly. It involves giving your undivided attention to the details at hand, blocking out any distractions and staying completely absorbed in completing the task accurately.

Visual search is the process that comes into play when you're trying to find a missing shoe for your child. You start with a mental picture of what the shoe looks like – its size, colour, shape and any distinctive features. With this image in mind, you methodically scan the room, filtering out irrelevant objects and focusing on identifying the specific shoe among the clutter. This type of focused searching involves coordinating your visual attention and memory as you actively compare the details of each item you see against the mental image of the missing shoe until you locate it.

Voluntary or **reflexive shifting** of attention occurs when something unexpected, like the sound of the school bus arriving, catches your focus. In an instant, you move your attention away from what you were doing – perhaps packing a lunchbox – to something more urgent, like grabbing your child's backpack and making sure they're ready to leave. This quick change in focus involves two key actions: first, letting go of your current task, and then immediately directing your attention to what now needs to be done. It's an automatic and swift response to a change in the situation, allowing you to prioritise what's most important in the moment.

Attentional filtering is similar to ignoring background noise, like the TV or a phone ringing, while you are concentrating on helping your child with something important. It's about choosing to focus your mind only on what really matters at that moment and blocking out any distractions that aren't relevant. This skill helps you to stay on task, ensuring that outside sounds or other distractions don't pull your attention away from what you need to be doing.

Expectation is like getting the umbrella ready because you heard the weather forecast predict rain. It's about thinking ahead and preparing for what might happen, so you're not caught off guard. By planning for the possibility of rain, you make sure your child is dressed appropriately and has everything they need to stay dry. It's a way of being proactive, using what you know to get ready for the day ahead.

These elements of attention help you to navigate the morning routine smoothly, ensuring your child gets to school prepared and on time.

Attention is a key differentiator between Autism and ADHD. Inattention manifests as difficulty maintaining focus on tasks, becoming easily distracted, zoning out during conversations and losing interest once the novelty of a task wears off. This lack of sustained attention significantly impacts the ability to remain engaged and productive.

Attention in Autism

In individuals with Autism, the ability to maintain sustained and focused attention is often stronger than that of the general population. This means they can concentrate on tasks for longer periods without losing focus. Additionally, their visual search skills are typically better, likely due to enhanced perceptual processing rather than purely attention-related factors.

However, they may experience difficulties in shifting their attention and switching focus, both instinctively and voluntarily, in specific situations. This can make it challenging for them to disengage from one task and move to another, especially when the new task is not socially engaging. Despite these challenges, their ability to filter out irrelevant information remains intact, particularly in those without intellectual disabilities. This means they can effectively ignore distractions and focus on relevant tasks when needed. This highlights the ability to notice small details and to focus deeply on particular interests.

This intense focus is often seen as meticulous attention to detail in some, while in others it manifests as a deep preoccupation. When absorbed in a particular hobby or interest, their concentration becomes unwavering and fixed. This is because such behaviours, values, feelings and thoughts are ego-syntonic, meaning they are naturally aligned with their personal needs, goals and self-image, thus creating a sense of harmony between their actions and their inner self.

In Autism, if a person lacks interest in a task, they often choose not to engage with it. This disinterest is frequently mistaken for a lack of attention or focus. However, attention in Autism can be quite intense – remarkably fixed and unwavering, often accompanied by a profound attention to detail.

Indifference in Autism often presents as a seeming disconnection from the surrounding world, where an individual might appear unresponsive to social cues, disinterested in engaging with others, or unenthusiastic about activities that generally capture the attention of their peers. This perceived detachment is not due to a lack of awareness but rather a reflection of their unique way of navigating their inner landscape.

Autistic individuals often find comfort and fulfilment in familiar routines, specialised interests or solitary activities, rather than in the unpredictability of social interactions. Their indifference is not a deliberate disregard, nor it is inattention, but rather a natural inclination towards environments that offer consistency and a sense of security. For them, the external world's demands can feel overwhelming, confusing or less compelling compared to the clarity and depth they experience within their focused interests or sensory world.

Attention in ADHD

In individuals with ADHD, it's important to consider different types of attention and their respective challenges.

Sustained attention – the ability to maintain focus over a prolonged period – is often impaired in individuals with ADHD, making it difficult for them to stay engaged with long or monotonous tasks. This leads to frequent task-switching and incomplete projects.

Focused attention, which involves concentrating on a specific task while ignoring distractions, is another area where people with ADHD struggle, often resulting in them getting easily sidetracked by external stimuli.

Selective attention – the capacity to prioritise relevant stimuli while ignoring irrelevant ones – poses a significant challenge for those with ADHD. They may find it hard to filter out distractions, leading to difficulties in concentrating during conversations and missing key details.

Alternating attention – the ability to shift focus between different tasks – is also problematic, making it hard for individuals with ADHD to transition smoothly between activities, especially in multitasking environments.

Divided attention, which involves processing multiple sources of information simultaneously, is often compromised in individuals with ADHD. This can result in errors and omissions, such as struggling to listen and take notes at the same time.

Attentional filtering – the process of focusing on important information while ignoring background noise – is impaired, leading to heightened sensitivity to environmental distractions and making it challenging to concentrate in noisy settings.

Interestingly, individuals with ADHD can experience periods of **hyperfocus**, when there is a pressing need or a significant deadline, even if the task is not inherently interesting.

These attentional difficulties significantly impact daily functioning in academic, professional and social settings. Understanding these challenges can inform better management strategies, such as using structured routines, minimising distractions and employing time-management techniques to improve focus and productivity.

2. Distraction vs Sensory Overload

> **Case Study 3:** Dylan, a nineteen-year-old university student with Autism, frequently experiences sensory overload due to heightened sensitivity to auditory, visual and tactile stimuli. This overload leads to distraction, anxiety and a need to escape from environments like lecture halls and libraries, impacting his academic performance and social interactions. To manage these challenges, Dylan uses sensory tools, plans his routine to avoid overwhelming settings and practises mindfulness, but these strategies also lead to social isolation and missed opportunities.

> **Case Study 4:** Sophia, a fourteen-year-old student with ADHD, predominantly inattentive type, faces significant challenges with distractibility in the classroom, affecting her academic performance. Easily sidetracked by noises, visuals or minor movements, she often misses important instructions and lesson content, leading to confusion and incomplete work. Despite showing good understanding when focused, her frequent

lapses disrupt both her individual learning and group activities. She was eventually referred by her SENCO for an ADHD assessment and was diagnosed.

Sensory Overload in Autism

In Autism, distractions are predominantly sensory in nature. Children with Autism are often overwhelmed by sensory stimuli, significantly hampering their ability to focus. Sounds that might seem ordinary to others – such as someone chewing or the crinkling of a bag of chips – can be intensely distracting and even unbearable. Background noises that go unnoticed by most, like the hum of electricity, the beeping of devices or the high-pitched frequencies of animal deterrents, can dominate their attention. At times, these heightened sensory experiences are so vivid that they are mistaken for hallucinations.

These sensory distractions are not limited to just sounds. They can also include overpowering scents, such as the smell of someone's breath, or visual stimuli like bright, glaring lights. Even tactile experiences, such as the sensation of someone sitting too close, can be overwhelming. The impact of this sensory overload goes beyond mere distraction; it can be profoundly distressing, leading those with Autism to avoid these environments whenever possible, in order to protect themselves from discomfort and anxiety.

Conversely, individuals with Autism might exhibit intense focus on specific interests or activities to the exclusion of other stimuli. This can make them appear distracted from tasks not related to their interests.

People with Autism can get distracted because it's hard for them to understand social cues and keep up with conversations, which can feel very overwhelming.

As they mature, adults with Autism often develop a variety of strategies to manage their sensory sensitivities and navigate a world that can feel overwhelmingly chaotic. These coping mechanisms are carefully crafted over time, allowing them to create a sense of predictability and control in their daily lives. Many rely on structured routines that help to minimise unexpected sensory input and reduce anxiety.

To shield themselves from sensory overload they might use noise-cancelling headphones that block out intrusive sounds, creating a personal bubble of calm amid the noise. Others may choose to work from home, where they can regulate their environment more effectively, away from the unpredictable stimuli of a busy office or public space. Some find comfort in dimly lit or dark rooms, where the absence of harsh lighting provides a reprieve for their overstimulated senses. Avoiding environments filled with strong smells, such as crowded restaurants or public transport, is another way they manage to maintain their equilibrium.

These adaptations are more than mere preferences; they are essential tools that allow adults with Autism to engage with the world on their own terms, ensuring they can function and thrive without being constantly overwhelmed by sensory input.

Distraction in ADHD

Imagine attempting to concentrate on a monotonous task, yet your mind continuously drifts away, drawn to a myriad of distractions – perhaps the sound of people talking nearby, a cascade of your own thoughts or a captivating event unfolding around you. In these moments, zoning out becomes a form of distraction, a gateway through which the mind escapes from the mundane. This wandering attention is constantly on the lookout for something more stimulating, something that promises novelty and excitement.

Distraction, in this sense, becomes a conduit for the restless mind to seek out the next intriguing or engaging thing, abandoning the current task for something that might provide a quicker, more gratifying hit of interest or reward. This relentless search for stimulation is at the heart of ADHD, where the mind's tendency to shift away from dull or repetitive activities is not just a fleeting habit but a defining characteristic. It reflects a deep-seated need for dynamism and novelty, making it challenging to stay tethered to any one task for long.

Distraction is driven by a craving for bursts of dopamine, the brain's reward chemical that provides a sense of pleasure and motivation. When one activity starts to lose its appeal or challenge, the mind seeks out the next captivating thing, lured by the promise of another dopamine rush. This cycle of sidetracking and seeking fresh stimulation is a restless search for satisfaction, where attention flits from one point of interest to another, never lingering long enough to complete a task but always seeking the next source of excitement and reward.

There's a flip side called hyperfocus. This intense focus is powerful but unpredictable and doesn't last long; it is driven by need, stress and incentivisation, unlike the consistent interests seen in people with Autism.

Executive functions, such as skills involving organisation, planning and prioritisation, present another significant challenge. For someone with ADHD, managing long-term projects or intricate tasks can feel like an overwhelming act of juggling too many balls at once. This often results in frustration and a trail of unfinished work, as the mind is easily lured away by distractions that offer a brief burst of novelty. However, this novelty is fleeting, prompting further shifts in focus and creating a cycle of continuous distraction.

In the context of ADHD, distractions stem largely from difficulties with sustained attention, especially when faced with tasks that lack inherent interest. Maintaining focus on such non-engaging activities becomes a constant struggle. To combat this, individuals with ADHD may employ strategies like using timers, creating lists or taking scheduled breaks to help anchor their attention and manage their focus more effectively.

3. No Filter vs Factual Discourse

> **Case Study 5:** Lily, a thirteen-year-old girl diagnosed with Autism, is characterised by her strong preference for factual discourse and a tendency to speak without a filter. At school Lily's impressive memory and ability to recall specific details and facts stand out, but her communication often lacks social nuance. She tends to state facts bluntly and literally, regardless of the social context or the feelings of those around her. For instance, during classroom discussions, if a fellow pupil gives an incorrect answer or misstates a fact, Lily immediately corrects them in a direct and sometimes abrupt manner, which

can be perceived as rude or dismissive. Her focus on accuracy over social sensitivity means that she frequently misses cues about when it might be more tactful to remain silent or soften her approach, leading to misunderstandings and occasional conflicts with classmates.

This 'no filter' style of communication extends to Lily's social interactions outside the classroom, where her bluntness can create barriers to forming close relationships. When engaging in conversations, she often focuses intensely on her areas of interest, such as scientific facts or historical events, and presents information in a very straightforward way, without consideration for the social dynamics at play. For example, if a friend is discussing a personal experience, Lily might interrupt to provide a fact that she deems relevant but that could come across as insensitive or unrelated to the emotional context. Her candid remarks and direct manner, while not intended to be hurtful, can sometimes alienate peers who may feel she lacks empathy or understanding.

Case Study 6: Mia, a sixteen-year-old with ADHD, predominantly combined presentation, exhibits a pronounced tendency to speak without a filter – a common characteristic of impulsivity in ADHD. This behaviour manifests itself in both her academic and social settings, where she often blurts out thoughts, jokes or critiques without considering the social context or potential impact on others. In the classroom, Mia's impulsive comments can disrupt lessons and offend peers, as she might suddenly interrupt to share unrelated stories or bluntly critique

> others' work. Similarly, in social situations, her unfiltered remarks such as commenting abruptly on a friend's appearance often lead to misunderstandings and strain her relationships.

To the casual observer, both Autism and ADHD may seem like a lack of filter, allowing thoughts or behaviours to flow without restraint. While this might look similar on the surface, the underlying reasons for these expressions are entirely distinct, shaped by the unique characteristics of each condition.

Factual Discourse in Autism

People with Autism say things as they see it. They are exceedingly factual, often expressing themselves with a bluntness that lacks concern for how their words might be received. If someone takes offence, they are unlikely to feel regret and are more inclined to assert that they are simply stating a fact.

What they express may indeed be a straightforward fact, their perspective on a situation or a reflection of their personal experiences, but to the listener it can sometimes appear as though the person lacks a filter or social tact. However, what may seem like a blunt or tactless interaction often stems from their commitment to being precise and honest in their communication.

An autistic individual is often perplexed as to why others might take offence at what they perceive to be a simple statement of fact. People with Autism frequently struggle with understanding social norms and cues, which can result in statements or actions that appear abrupt or inappropriate because they are not attuned to social expectations.

The lack of a filter in Autism is usually due to a genuine difficulty in recognising what is socially acceptable or expected. For example, an autistic person might make a direct comment about someone's appearance without realising it could be hurtful, simply because they do not grasp the social subtleties involved.

No Filter in ADHD

Individuals with ADHD often lack a filter due to the impulsive nature of the condition. They may speak or act without thinking, driven by an inability to control their immediate reactions. This impulsivity frequently leads to blurting out thoughts or interrupting conversations, as they struggle to pause and consider the appropriateness of their words. They are reflective of their experiences but, due to impulsivity, may do it again.

The impulsivity associated with ADHD affects executive functioning, which includes self-control. As a result, individuals might find it challenging to stop themselves from vocalising thoughts the moment they arise. While they may recognise that certain statements are inappropriate, the lack of impulse control prevents them from inhibiting these reactions. This behaviour stems from impulsivity rather than a lack of social understanding, distinguishing it from other conditions where social cues and norms are not well understood.

Autism:	The lack of filter is generally due to a genuine difficulty in understanding social norms and subtleties, leading to direct and sometimes blunt communication.

ADHD: The lack of filter stems from impulsivity and poor self-control, leading to spontaneous and often inappropriate comments or actions despite understanding social norms.

4. Hyperfocus vs Preoccupation

Case Study 7: Jake, a twenty-one-year-old university student with ADHD, predominantly inattentive type, often procrastinates on assignments, leading to intense episodes of hyperfocus when facing last-minute deadlines. One example of this pattern occurred during his final semester, when he delayed a major design project until the last twenty-four hours. The looming deadline triggered a hyperfocus response, where Jake became fully engrossed in his work, blocking out all distractions and working non-stop. While this allowed him to produce high-quality work, it came at the cost of sleep, nutrition and overall well-being, affecting his performance in other areas.

Case Study 8: Sarah, a thirty-four-year-old policewoman with Autism, has a deep preoccupation with building a detailed Lego city – a focused interest and creative outlet that provides her with relaxation and a sense of control.

Sarah's fascination with Lego began in childhood but grew into an intense hobby in adulthood, resulting in the construction of a vast, intricate Lego city that occupies a significant portion of her attic. Her city is meticulously planned, featuring detailed buildings, transport networks and realistic cityscapes, all of

> which she builds and organises with extraordinary precision. After long and demanding shifts at the police station, Sarah often retreats to her attic, where she spends hours constructing new sections, redesigning layouts and meticulously arranging every element of her Lego city. This preoccupation is so absorbing that Sarah often loses track of time, missing meals, neglecting household chores and experiencing distress if she is interrupted or asked to leave her project. This intense focus affects her social interactions and work-life balance, as she frequently steers conversations towards her Lego hobby and prefers solitary time over social activities.

Hyperfocus is a powerful state where the brain seeks dopamine, particularly in moments of low motivation or during episodes of procrastination. This intense concentration is often triggered by deep interests, looming deadlines or high-stress situations. It is maintained through a scaffolding of strategies and routines that support sustained attention. Individuals in a state of hyperfocus are acutely aware that any interruption could disrupt their flow, making it challenging to re-engage with the task at hand once they stop.

In writing about AuDHD, it is essential to acknowledge the profound depth of preoccupation seen in individuals. Their intense focus on a particular topic, field or set of facts stems from a genuine passion and an innate love for that area of expertise. This fascination drives an unquenchable desire to gather more knowledge, often leading them to accumulate information surpassing even that of recognised experts.

Such preoccupations can vary in duration – they might captivate the individual for a few months or persist for years, or even a lifetime. The excitement and joy they derive from this deep dive into their interests are palpable, fuelling their commitment and enthusiasm. Whether these interests are transient or enduring, the knowledge they acquire is both comprehensive and detailed, showcasing their remarkable capacity for focused learning and expertise.

Preoccupation in Autism

Individuals with Autism often develop intense interests in various fields, such as science and technology. This can lead to a deep fascination with subjects like astronomy, biology or physics. They dedicate significant time to reading, researching and experimenting, often gaining more knowledge than peers or professionals. For example, an individual might become an expert in astrophysics, mastering complex theories and phenomena due to their relentless curiosity and passion.

Collecting items and data is another common interest among autistic individuals. They may collect stamps, coins or other items, organising and cataloguing them with incredible precision. This hobby can extend to creating comprehensive databases about their collections. For example, a person might meticulously document a vast collection of stamps from around the world, providing a sense of structure and satisfaction.

Autistic individuals often develop hobbies and skills requiring a high degree of expertise, such as model building, cooking or sports. Their approach is methodical and detail-oriented. For example, someone might spend years perfecting their culinary ability or becoming exceptionally skilled in a sport, understanding every rule and technique. These hobbies provide enjoyment and a way to channel their focus and energy.

The duration and intensity of these preoccupations can vary widely. Some interests might be short-lived, while others can persist for years or a lifetime. For example, a young person might be fascinated by dinosaurs for several years before shifting to a new interest. Conversely, someone might maintain a lifelong passion for classical music, continuously expanding their knowledge.

Special interests in Autism provide comfort, structure and predictability, helping to manage anxiety and sensory overload. Engaging with their interests provides a sense of control and accomplishment, though these intense preoccupations can also lead to difficulties in social interactions and flexibility. Juggling these interests with broader engagement in life can be challenging, but it's crucial for a fulfilling and balanced life.

Recognising and supporting these special interests is vital. Encouraging their exploration and development can lead to significant personal growth. At the same time, fostering social skills and broader engagement with the world is essential. This might involve integrating interests into social and educational settings, as well as helping individuals to navigate and balance different aspects of life. For example, a teacher might use a student's interest in trains to connect with classmates and learn other subjects through their passion.

By understanding and supporting these interests, we can help individuals with Autism lead enriched, balanced lives, leveraging their passions while fostering broader social and personal development.

Hyperfocus in ADHD

ADHD can be described as an insatiable quest for constant stimulation.

Hyperfocus in ADHD is commonly associated with tasks or activities that the individual finds particularly interesting or stimulating, or that offer a high level of immediate gratification. This intense concentration allows them to become deeply engrossed in these activities, often losing track of time and ignoring other important tasks or responsibilities.

For instance, an individual with ADHD might hyperfocus on video games, which are a constant source of stimulation, and find them intrinsically motivating. This focus can be so intense that they become unaware of their surroundings or the passage of time, sometimes to the detriment of necessary activities like eating or sleeping.

Hyperfocus can also occur in situations where there is a pressing need or a significant deadline, even if the task is not inherently interesting. The urgency and pressure to complete the task can trigger a hyperfocused state as a coping mechanism to deal with the impending deadline.

While hyperfocus can be beneficial in allowing individuals with ADHD to accomplish complex tasks and delve deeply into subjects they are passionate about, it also highlights the challenge of managing attention and balancing various responsibilities. Developing strategies to manage hyperfocus, such as setting timers, creating schedules and employing reminders, can help individuals with ADHD navigate their daily activities more effectively.

Overall, hyperfocus in ADHD is primarily driven by interest and stimulation, but it can also be influenced by urgency and necessity in certain situations. This dual nature underscores the complexity of attentional regulation in individuals with ADHD.

5. Social Inappropriateness vs Social Awkwardness

Case Study 9: Helen, a forty-five-year-old accountant recently diagnosed with Autism, faces significant challenges related to social awkwardness, impacting her personal and professional life. Despite her intelligence and success at work, Helen often struggles to read social cues like facial expressions, tone of voice and body language, leading to frequent misunderstandings. In professional settings, she may interrupt conversations without realising it or dominate discussions with topics of personal interest, which some colleagues perceive as abrupt or self-centred. In social gatherings, she often feels out of place, finding it difficult to engage in small talk or follow the flow of conversations, which leaves her feeling isolated and unsure of how to connect with others.

Helen's social difficulties also affect her personal relationships, where her literal thinking and focus on factual details can lead to misinterpretations and create emotional distance. For example, she may respond seriously to jokes or figurative language, missing the intended humour or context.

Case Study 10: Alex, a twenty-seven-year-old non-binary individual with ADHD, predominantly combined presentation, faces challenges with social appropriateness due to impulsivity and difficulties with self-regulation. Known for their creativity and enthusiasm, they often struggle to navigate social norms, leading to misunderstandings in both personal and professional settings. At their job in a marketing firm, they frequently interrupt colleagues during meetings to share ideas, sometimes going off-topic or dominating conversations. While their contributions can be valuable, the timing and delivery often come across as inappropriate or disruptive. They may also make blunt comments or jokes without realising these might be perceived as insensitive or out of place, resulting in frustration among coworkers.

Outside of work, their impulsive behaviour affects their social life, where they might overshare personal details or ask intrusive questions without recognising the discomfort these could cause. At a recent gathering, they discussed a friend's relationship issues in front of others, not understanding that doing so could breach social boundaries. This often leaves them feeling isolated, as they struggle to understand why their interactions sometimes lead to tension.

People often label individuals with Autism and ADHD as lacking social skills or being socially awkward. This broad categorisation overlooks the complexities of their social experiences and interactions. It fails to recognise that the social challenges faced by those with Autism or ADHD are not due to a lack of desire for connection but are often rooted in the distinct ways they perceive, process and respond to social cues. Such assumptions simplify the nuanced realities of their social behaviours, which are shaped by different neurological patterns and sensory experiences rather than an inherent inability to engage socially.

Social Awkwardness in Autism

Social awkwardness in Autism is characterised by various distinct behaviours stemming from challenges in understanding and responding to social cues. One key aspect is eye contact; many autistic individuals find it difficult to maintain, often resulting in either avoidance or fleeting eye contact, which others might misinterpret as disinterest or evasiveness.

Understanding social norms is another challenge, as autistic individuals may struggle to grasp and adhere to these conventions. This can lead to behaviours that seem unusual or inappropriate in social settings, such as difficulty initiating or sustaining conversations, or speaking bluntly without considering the context.

In new or unexpected social situations, social awkwardness becomes especially pronounced. The unpredictability of these scenarios can cause significant anxiety, making it hard for autistic individuals to know how to act, what to say or how to behave. This uncertainty often results in visible discomfort and heightened self-consciousness.

Additionally, autistic individuals might prefer solitude to large gatherings or social events. The overwhelming sensory input and social demands in such settings can be exhausting, prompting them to seek solitude to manage their anxiety and stress.

Difficulties with non-verbal communication are also common. Autistic individuals might struggle to interpret body language, facial expressions and tone of voice, making it challenging to understand others' emotions and intentions. Conversely, their own non-verbal cues might not align with their spoken words, causing further misunderstandings.

Lastly, engaging in the give-and-take of social interactions can be difficult. Autistic individuals might dominate conversations with topics of personal interest, miss social cues indicating that others want to speak, or lack the knowledge of how to engage in small talk. These behaviours can lead to perceptions of social awkwardness or aloofness.

Social Inappropriateness in ADHD

Individuals with ADHD often grapple with a variety of social difficulties that stem from the core symptoms of inattention, hyperactivity and impulsivity. These challenges significantly impact their ability to form and maintain social relationships.

Firstly, impulsivity can cause individuals with ADHD to frequently interrupt others during conversations, as they struggle to wait their turn to speak. This behaviour is often perceived as rude or disrespectful, leading to social friction. Additionally, they might blurt out inappropriate comments without considering the social context, resulting in misunderstandings or hurt feelings.

Inattention presents another set of challenges. People with ADHD often find it difficult to sustain focus during conversations, which can lead to missed social cues or an appearance of disinterest. They are easily distracted by their surroundings, making it hard to maintain consistent and engaging interactions with others.

Hyperactivity further complicates social interactions. The physical restlessness common in ADHD can be off-putting in social settings, as constant movement or fidgeting may signal impatience or a lack of interest. Their need to be constantly active can overwhelm peers, making integration into group activities or discussions difficult. They might get up in meetings or take several breaks during the day for tea. As children, they would get up from their seats, run around and take bathroom breaks even when they didn't need it.

Moreover, individuals with ADHD often struggle with misinterpretation that can lead to inappropriate reactions and difficulty responding appropriately in social situations, exacerbating social awkwardness.

Those with ADHD frequently experience emotions more intensely and may have trouble controlling these emotions, leading to overreactions to social stimuli. Frequent mood swings add to this challenge, making it hard for peers to predict reactions and potentially resulting in social isolation.

Forming and maintaining friendships can be particularly challenging. The variability in behaviour driven by ADHD symptoms can make it hard to maintain consistent and stable relationships. Additionally, in group settings, individuals with ADHD might struggle with cooperation and adherence to group norms, which can hinder the development of friendships. They then move from one friendship group to another, and often have rifts due to their impulsive behaviours.

6. Over-Talkativeness vs Talking Passionately

There is often a simplistic perception that individuals with ADHD are excessively talkative and loud, while those with Autism are reserved and quiet. This view paints a picture of ADHD as a constant flurry of words and energy – individuals who speak rapidly, their conversations marked by tangents and an eagerness to share whatever is on their mind. They may seem to fill the room with their presence, animated by the thoughts rushing through their heads, unable to contain their excitement or impulse to speak.

Conversely, people with Autism are frequently stereotyped as the silent observers in the room, the ones who speak less and prefer to listen or simply withdraw. They are seen as inwardly focused, communicating sparingly and often only when necessary. Their quietness is mistaken for shyness, detachment or a lack of interest in engaging with others.

> **Case Study 11:** John, a thirty-five-year-old software engineer with ADHD, predominantly combined presentation, struggles with over-talkativeness – a trait commonly associated with ADHD-related impulsivity and hyperactivity. In professional settings, John often dominates conversations during meetings or collaborative projects, speaking at length about his ideas and technical details. While his knowledge and enthusiasm are appreciated, his tendency to speak without noticing when others wish to contribute can hinder balanced discussions. This has led to some coworkers feeling overshadowed or excluded during meetings, impacting team dynamics and collaboration.
>
> In social situations, John's over-talkativeness similarly creates challenges in forming deeper connections. He frequently misses cues that others want to speak or that a topic has become tiresome, which can come across as self-centred or inconsiderate, even though he is unaware of this perception. Friends and family sometimes avoid group settings

with him, concerned they won't have the chance to engage in conversation.

Case Study 12: Linda, a fifty-two-year-old woman recently diagnosed with Autism, has a unique communication style: she speaks passionately and at length about her favourite topics, such as classical literature, environmental science and ancient history. Outside of these interests, Linda is generally not very talkative and tends to be reserved. However, when discussing her areas of expertise, she becomes highly animated, often going into deep detail and speaking for extended periods without noticing if others are engaged or ready to change the topic. This intense focus on specific subjects can sometimes overwhelm her listeners, leading to feelings of disconnection or frustration in social settings, as they may struggle to contribute to the conversation.

Understanding her recent Autism diagnosis has provided Linda with clarity about why she has always found it challenging to gauge social cues or adjust her speech accordingly. This newfound awareness is helping her to recognise the need for a more balanced approach in her interactions.

Talking Passionately in Autism

Over-talkativeness in Autism, often referred to as 'hyper-verbal' communication, manifests in several unique ways; it is primarily driven by an intense interest in specific topics, challenges in understanding social cues, and a tendency towards detailed and literal communication.

Individuals with Autism often have deep, intense interests in specific subjects. When engaged in a conversation about these topics, they can become extremely talkative, sharing extensive details and information, which they find comforting, especially in social situations where they feel anxious or uncertain. Their enthusiasm can lead to prolonged monologues, as a way to navigate social interactions more comfortably. They might not recognise the social norms of turn-taking in conversations, leading to one-sided discussions where they do most of the talking. This can result in them dominating conversations without realising they are not giving others a chance to contribute.

Communication in Autism tends to be very literal and detailed. When asked a question, they might provide exhaustive information rather than summarising. The passion and enthusiasm for their interests drive autistic individuals to share information with great fervour. This can come across as over-talkativeness, but it is rooted in a genuine desire to communicate and connect over topics they care deeply about.

Over-Talkativeness in ADHD

Individuals with ADHD mostly love to talk, take over a conversation, change its themes very quickly and, yes, they don't get the cue that the other person might be getting bored. They are loud in social interactions and generally seen as the heart and soul of the party.

They may feel an urgent need to share their thoughts immediately, leading to frequent interruptions during conversations. This impulsivity makes it difficult for them to wait their turn to speak, often resulting in talking over others.

People with ADHD may speak rapidly, trying to convey their thoughts as quickly as they materialise. This can lead to overloading listeners with information and making it challenging for others to follow the conversation. The rapid pace of speech is often a reflection of their racing thoughts and the need to express them quickly, before they are lost or forgotten. Over-talkativeness in ADHD can also be linked to challenges with active listening.

The tendency to talk excessively can impact social relationships. It may lead to frustration or annoyance in others, who might feel unheard or overshadowed in conversations. Over time, this can strain friendships and professional relationships if not addressed.

7. Impulsivity vs Acting Out

> **Case Study 13:** Maria is a forty-eight-year-old woman recently diagnosed with Autism. She exhibits impulsive behaviours that significantly affect her daily life and social interactions. While she is highly intelligent and has a successful career as a graphic designer, Maria often struggles with impulsivity, particularly in social and professional contexts. She often acts or speaks without considering the consequences or the social appropriateness of her actions. For instance, during work meetings she frequently interrupts colleagues to share her thoughts or new ideas, sometimes completely changing the subject or focusing on details that others may not find relevant. This tendency to speak out of turn can create tension among her coworkers, who may perceive her as rude or overly direct, even though she

does not intend to offend. In social settings Maria may abruptly change plans, make spontaneous decisions without consulting others or make blunt comments that can be perceived as insensitive. For example, she once invited a group of friends over for dinner without checking if they were available, assuming they would adapt to her plan, which led to confusion and hurt feelings.

Case Study 14: Salman, a twenty-year-old Pakistani male diagnosed with Attention Deficit Hyperactivity Disorder (ADHD), predominantly combined presentation, exhibits significant impulsivity that has led to a range of challenges in his personal and social life. Unemployed and struggling to manage daily responsibilities, Salman's impulsive behaviour has resulted in conflicts with law enforcement, recreational substance use, financial debt and frequent involvement in physical altercations.

Salman has a long history of impulsive behaviour, a core characteristic of his ADHD, which has worsened since he left school. Lacking stable employment, he often acts on immediate urges without considering the potential outcomes. His impulsivity leads him to spend money recklessly, accumulating substantial debt from impulsive purchases and gambling, often borrowing money without thinking about how he will repay it. Additionally, Salman has started using recreational substances like marijuana, cocaine and alcohol, which further impair his judgment and increase his risk-taking behaviours. He often gets into trouble with the police for public disturbances, petty theft or being caught in possession of illegal substances.

> Salman's impulsivity also manifests in his frequent involvement in fights, usually triggered by minor disagreements or perceived slights when he is under the influence of substances or in highly stimulating environments like bars or clubs. His inability to control his temper or consider the consequences often leads to escalation and physical confrontations.

We often associate impulsivity with people who have ADHD, but it's important to recognise that individuals with Autism can also be described as impulsive.

Impulsivity in Autism

Impulsivity in Autism is influenced by various factors, including sensory sensitivities, communication challenges, and the need for routine and predictability.

Autistic individuals often exhibit heightened sensitivity to sensory input, which can trigger impulsive behaviours. For instance, an overwhelming sound or a sudden change in light can lead to immediate, unplanned reactions, such as covering ears or fleeing the scene. These responses are not premeditated, but rather instinctive attempts to manage sensory overload.

Communication challenges also play a significant role. An autistic person might impulsively interrupt conversations or speak out of turn because they struggle to grasp the social cues that govern the flow of dialogue. Their need to express themselves immediately can override social norms, resulting in impulsive speech.

The necessity for routine and predictability is a core aspect of Autism. When routines are disrupted, it can cause significant stress, leading to impulsive actions as the individual seeks to regain a sense of control. This need for order and consistency drives their behaviour, particularly in unpredictable situations.

Moreover, autistic individuals might react impulsively to emotional stimuli, displaying sudden outbursts of anger, joy or frustration without typical social filters. These reactions are often responses to immediate emotional needs rather than calculated actions.

Recognising the unique triggers and manifestations of impulsivity in Autism is crucial for caregivers and educators. By understanding these differences, they can create more supportive environments that accommodate these needs and help to manage impulsive behaviours effectively. This approach not only mitigates impulsivity, but also fosters a more inclusive and understanding atmosphere for autistic individuals.

Impulsivity in ADHD

Impulsivity can take so many forms: the impulsive nature of ADHD can lead to a higher propensity for risk-taking behaviours like binge eating, gambling, using recreational substances or putting oneself in harm's way and others, too.

This impulsivity entails high risks and generally has to be curbed.

People with ADHD often prefer immediate rewards over delayed ones. This difficulty in delaying gratification can lead to challenges in setting and achieving long-term goals, as they may opt for short-term gains instead.

Impulsivity affects decision-making processes, leading individuals to make hasty decisions without thoroughly evaluating options or potential outcomes. This can result in poor choices that have negative repercussions.

In conversations, impulsive individuals may blurt out responses or comments without considering whether it is their turn to speak or their input is relevant.

Impulsivity can significantly impact academic or work performance, especially in situations requiring sustained attention and careful planning. This tendency to act hastily without thorough consideration often leads to errors and reduces overall productivity. I have seen very smart people unable to complete their education or do it too late in their lives. They also are unable to hold jobs for long, impulsively leaving employment when the novelty is over.

Impulsivity is fuelled by a craving for novelty, a pursuit of quick dopamine bursts that can be triggered by thrill-seeking adventures, daredevil stunts, or the adrenaline rush of stealing for the sheer excitement of it. This restless search for stimulation often leads to entanglements with the criminal justice system, as the boundaries between risk and recklessness blur. The use of recreational substances is another manifestation of this impulsivity, as it reflects a constant desire to chase new sensations and escape the ordinary.

In the next chapter, we will delve into the complex and fascinating presentation of AuDHD, a term that encapsulates the co-occurrence of Autism and Attention Deficit Hyperactivity Disorder (ADHD). This exploration will address why we are witnessing a sudden surge in AuDHD diagnoses, as well as offering a comprehensive understanding of this dual diagnosis and its management.

Chapter 5: The Rise of AuDHD

In secondary school, after a parent-teacher meeting, my parents and I were heading home. I had placed second in my class overall, but my parents had hoped I would maintain the top position, as I had in previous exams. My performance, however, had become unpredictable – sometimes excellent, sometimes not – without any clear reason. As we drove, my father (may he rest in peace) turned to me and said, 'You're so consistently inconsistent.' I paused, gathered my thoughts, and then replied, 'But, Dad, isn't that a kind of consistency?' He was silent for a moment, then grinned. And that, in a nutshell, is how AuDHD operates.

The recent increase in AuDHD diagnoses can be largely attributed to changes in how mental health professionals recognise and diagnose both Autism and ADHD together. Before 2013, it was not possible for someone to be officially diagnosed with both autism and ADHD. If a person was diagnosed with one, they simply couldn't be diagnosed with the other. This changed when the *Diagnostic and Statistical Manual of Mental Disorders* (DSM-5) was updated in 2013. The new criteria allowed for the acknowledgment that a person can have both Autism and ADHD, leading to more accurate diagnoses and an increase in identified cases of AuDHD.

Even though AuDHD is not an official diagnosis, professionals can now diagnose someone with both ADHD and Autism if they show signs of both, and if they meet the diagnosis based on DSM-5 or ICD-11. It takes an experienced professional to identify both conditions accurately because symptoms of one, as we've already seen, might overshadow the other. Recognising both conditions is crucial because they impact daily life in different ways.

Many individuals with AuDHD describe their experience as akin to having split personalities, reminiscent of Dr Jekyll and Mr Hyde. They often feel as though their minds are divided, embodying contradictions that constantly shift and change. During assessments, people often share a sense of persistent confusion, recognising traits of both conditions as they oscillate between them. This dynamic interplay is like a seesaw, presenting in three distinct ways: in some, Autism is more prominent than ADHD; in others, ADHD features dominate over those of Autism. Then there are cases where the prominence of Autism and ADHD fluctuates, with one sometimes overshadowing the other and vice versa. This variability underscores the complexity of living with both conditions, highlighting the need for nuanced understanding and tailored support.

> **Case Study 1 ADHD Dominant AuDHD:** Serena was a thirty-year-old single, unemployed woman from a Southeast Asian background, referred for an ADHD assessment. Coming from a family with a history of neurodiversity, including a sister diagnosed with Autism, she exhibited lifelong symptoms such as a lack of attention span, poor organisation, forgetfulness, fidgetiness and impulsive behaviours. During

our session, I carried a laptop and, in my usual clumsy manner, its battery fell on the desk with a loud bang. The noise startled her noticeably. This happened again a few minutes later, eliciting a similarly strong response. These reactions seemed disproportionately intense compared to the stimuli, indicating distress from sensory overload. As the assessment continued, I also observed her fleeting eye contact and very literal speech. These observations prompted me to explore her history further, leading to a high score on the Autism triage. She was referred for an Autism assessment and diagnosed with ADHD Combined Type. If it hadn't been for her pronounced startled responses drawing my attention to other Autism-related traits, her Autism might have remained undiagnosed.

Case Study 2 Autism Dominant AuDHD: Samuel was a thirty-nine-year-old Caucasian male referred for an Autism assessment due to long-standing difficulties in social interaction, reciprocal communication, initiating conversations, making and sustaining friendships, and responding severely to changes and sensory overload. He had a deep interest in space and collected memorabilia

During the assessment, I observed his fidgetiness and restlessness, initially mistaking these movements for stimming. However, his actions were not repetitive but rather involved leg bouncing and fidgeting with his hands. He shared that despite his discrete interests, he struggled to concentrate for long periods, was forgetful and frequently left things behind.

As the evaluation progressed, it became evident that he had persistent difficulties with attention span, organisation and forgetfulness, which had progressively worsened over time. Socially, he avoided gatherings, preferred his own company, found small talk pointless, never had any friends, and reacted very negatively to change. He needed time to prepare for changes and desired to be organised but found it challenging. Ultimately, he was diagnosed with ADHD after initially being diagnosed with Autism.

Case Study 3 Variable AuDHD: Eleanor was a fifty-eight-year-old Caucasian woman referred for an ADHD assessment. She confessed that she had been postponing this assessment for the past thirty years, struggling to understand the dichotomy in her behaviour. On one hand, she exhibited exceptional organisational skills in certain areas, while in others she was strikingly disorganised. Her attention span showed similar contradictions, with an intense focus on some tasks and complete inattentiveness towards others. She described a constant oscillation between ADHD and autistic traits – a pattern that had perplexed her for decades. She had consulted at least a dozen psychiatrists over the years without finding clarity. As she recounted her experiences, I couldn't help but smile. Curious, she asked why I was smiling, and I responded that I might finally be able to explain the root of her struggles. After thoroughly assessing her symptoms, I diagnosed her with ADHD and highlighted the autistic features that contributed to her challenges. Upon receiving this feedback and finally understanding the interplay between her ADHD and Autism, she burst into tears. This diagnosis offered her a profound sense of relief and validation, helping her to make sense of the complexities that had defined her life for so long.

Autism and ADHD in AuDHD

1. Organisation vs Disorganisation

Disorganisation in ADHD

In my work as a neurodivergent psychiatrist, I often encounter patients who express a deep yearning for organisation yet find themselves unable to achieve it. This sentiment echoes across many of my assessments. Some individuals with ADHD exhibit profound challenges with attention, distractibility, procrastination and task completion, yet maintain immaculate organisational skills. They are never late, never lose or misplace things, and always put items in their proper place. In these cases, I frequently uncover Autism lurking beneath the ADHD.

Ego-Dystonic and Ego-Syntonic Attributes in Organisation

Understanding this dichotomy requires a closer examination of organisational tendencies. In ADHD, organisational skills often serve as a scaffolding – a support structure implemented out of necessity. ADHD individuals recognise that without these structures, their lives would descend into chaos and disarray. This type of organisation is ego-dystonic, meaning it conflicts with the individual's self-perception, values and beliefs. These behaviours are perceived as distressing, inappropriate and inconsistent with their identity, feeling like a burdensome imposition.

Conversely, when organisation is instinctual and there is a genuine love for orderliness, it typically indicates underlying Autism. Autistic individuals might spend hours meticulously organising, driven by an inherent need for structure and predictability. This form of organisation is ego-syntonic, meaning it aligns with the individual's self-image and values. The person perceives these behaviours as acceptable, appropriate and consistent with their identity.

This distinction between ego-syntonic and ego-dystonic organisation helps in understanding the underlying dynamics of ADHD and Autism. It also guides the therapeutic approach, ensuring that interventions are tailored to the unique needs and experiences of everyone, fostering a better quality of life and greater self-understanding.

Spectrum of Organisation in AuDHD

In AuDHD, the concept of organisation resembles a delicate seesaw, balancing unique traits from both Autism and ADHD. On one side, Autism contributes an ego-syntonic organisation – one that aligns harmoniously with the individual's sense of self. On the other, ADHD introduces a duality: a disorganised chaos where life and thoughts may feel scattered, contrasted sharply by moments of rigid, ego-dystonic organisation. This strict order emerges as a coping mechanism to counterbalance the potential collapse of chaos, much like a precarious house of cards. However, Autism's inherent structure often tempers the anarchy of ADHD, preventing it from descending into complete disarray. Together, Autism and ADHD engage in a complex interplay, creating a dynamic balancing act that makes AuDHD's presentation unconventional and, at times, challenging to discern.

> **Case Study 4:** Sarah, a twenty-nine-year-old graphic designer with AuDHD, experiences a striking contrast between her highly organised work life and her disorganised personal life. At work, her autistic traits drive a love for structure and order, making her organisation feel natural and ego-syntonic. However, at home her ADHD dominates, leading to chaos and disarray, which she finds distressing and ego-dystonic, as it conflicts with her desire for order. This duality represents the spectrum of organisation in AuDHD, where Autism and ADHD engage in a balancing act, each influencing different aspects of her life. Therapeutic interventions must respect this interplay, helping Sarah to integrate strategies that align with her natural tendencies and support areas of disorganisation.

2. Silence vs Noise/Stimulation

Silence and Autism

Autism is about the fear of the unknown, the anxiety around it and wanting to know all the possibilities of a certain situation. Autism is often characterised by a profound need for predictability and a deep-seated anxiety about the unknown.

Overstimulation

This anxiety manifests as a desire to understand and anticipate all possible outcomes in each situation. It's about being comfortable in one's own skin, preferring to be in one's own company and sitting in silence with limited stimulation. Stimulation can be anything from being in a new situation, a new environment, a new place, a new job, a new project, new colleagues or new people. This could translate into unknown situations, unpredictable circumstances, sensory overload, change in circumstances and disruption of routines – hence a preference for silence in comparison to stimulation.

Autistic individuals tend to be most comfortable in their own company, where they can engage in activities without the stress of social interaction. This preference for solitude is not a sign of anti-social behaviour, but rather a mechanism to avoid overstimulation and anxiety. Silence and solitude provide a soothing environment where creativity and innovation can flourish without the disruptions of an unpredictable world.

New situations, environments and social interactions can be particularly challenging for those with Autism. The unpredictability of a new job, project or meeting new colleagues can lead to significant stress and sensory overload. These scenarios disrupt the carefully structured routines that provide a sense of stability and control. As a result, autistic individuals might avoid new experiences, preferring the predictability of familiar settings.

Sensory Overload

Sensory overload is a common experience for autistic individuals. New stimuli, whether it be sounds, lights or social interactions, can become overwhelming. This sensory overload, coupled with the anxiety of unpredictability, makes change and new experiences daunting.

Consequently, disruptions to their routines can be distressing, leading to a strong preference for quiet, controlled environments.

For many autistic individuals, silence is not synonymous with a lack of creativity or innovation. On the contrary, a quiet environment provides the ideal conditions for their creativity to thrive. The absence of external stimuli allows them to focus deeply, think critically and engage in innovative thinking.

ADHD and Stimulation

ADHD is characterised by a relentless need for stimulation to regulate norepinephrine and dopamine levels in the brain. This need for constant stimulation drives individuals with ADHD to seek new and exciting experiences to keep their brains engaged and balanced.

The brain of an individual with ADHD operates differently in terms of neurotransmitter regulation, particularly concerning norepinephrine and dopamine, which play a crucial role in attention, motivation and reward processing.

Novelty People with ADHD often find themselves drawn to novel experiences and activities. Whether it's trying a new food, taking up a new hobby, meeting a new partner, starting a new job, or engaging in spontaneous activities like shopping or sex, these experiences provide the necessary stimulation to keep their brains active and satisfied. This quest for newness helps to regulate the neurotransmitters that are often imbalanced in ADHD, particularly norepinephrine and dopamine.

This constant search for stimulation can lead to a pattern of acquiring multiple hobbies and interests, often sidetracking from one to another without fully committing to any single one. This can result in a trail of unfinished projects and a lack of follow-through on tasks. The initial excitement of a new challenge or opportunity is invigorating, but it can quickly wane, leading to a cycle of losing interest and seeking the next stimulating activity.

The Impact The undeterred quest for stimulation can affect various aspects of life, from personal relationships to professional responsibilities. The need to pursue an unachievable goal or the excitement of a new challenge can sometimes overshadow the importance of completing existing tasks. This can make it difficult for individuals with ADHD to maintain focus and productivity in their daily lives.

AuDHD – Silence vs Stimulation

In individuals with AuDHD, there is a unique interplay between the need for stimulation and the experience of autistic burnouts. The latter is a state of physical, mental and emotional exhaustion brought on by stress and the cumulative impact of environments that do not cater to an individual's needs. Social interactions and situations can rapidly drain physical and mental energy, leaving a person feeling depleted.

The ADHD component of AuDHD creates a strong desire for stimulation, driving individuals to engage in activities that provide excitement and novelty. These activities are often solitary, such as running, swimming or rock climbing, aligning with the autistic preference for less social engagement. These pursuits offer a boost of energy and confidence through the release of dopamine and norepinephrine.

However, once this energy is depleted, burnout can occur. This leads to situations where individuals initially enjoy social interactions but suddenly feel overwhelmed and need to withdraw. They find themselves loving the experience one moment, only to feel drained and disconnected the next, highlighting the complex relationship between their need for stimulation and the risk of burnout.

The Interplay In individuals with AuDHD there exists a fascinating interplay between the desire for stimulation driven by ADHD and the phenomenon of autistic burnout. This dynamic creates a unique experience that blends the characteristics of both Autism and ADHD, leading to cycles of intense activity followed by periods of exhaustion.

Components of AuDHD The ADHD component in AuDHD manifests as a persistent need for stimulation. This desire fuels engagement in various activities, often those that are physically or mentally demanding and usually solitary. Activities like running, swimming and rock climbing are common choices. These pursuits provide the necessary dopamine and norepinephrine boosts, enhancing energy levels and confidence, and offering a sense of fulfilment and achievement.

However, this heightened state of activity and engagement is often followed by autistic burnout. This is a state of physical, mental and emotional exhaustion that occurs due to prolonged stress and exposure to environments that do not cater to the individual's needs. Social interactions and stimulating activities can rapidly deplete energy reserves, leading to a significant drop in both physical and mental vitality.

Energy and Burnout This cycle of energy and burnout creates a dichotomy where individuals with AuDHD experience alternating periods of high energy and severe exhaustion. They may initially thrive in stimulating environments, gaining enjoyment and satisfaction from social interactions and engaging activities. However, as their energy depletes, they may find themselves overwhelmed and fatigued, needing to retreat from these situations to recover.

To manage this cycle, individuals with AuDHD often gravitate towards solitary activities that allow them to balance their need for stimulation with their need for recovery and self-regulation. Engaging in solitary pursuits helps them to avoid the sensory overload and social demands that contribute to burnout, providing a controlled environment where they can manage their energy levels more effectively.

This dynamic often results in a love-hate relationship with stimulating activities. On one hand, individuals with AuDHD are drawn to them for the mental engagement and pleasure they provide. On the other hand, the inevitable burnout that follows can lead to frustration and a need to withdraw. They love the thrill and fulfilment of engagement but are often forced to step back when the consequences of overexertion take their toll.

> **Case Study 5:** James, a thirty-four-year-old software engineer with AuDHD, navigates a complex balance between his autistic need for silence and

structure, and his ADHD-driven desire for stimulation. At work, he thrives in quiet, controlled environments, where routine and solitude allow him to excel. Outside of work he seeks quiet, nature-based activities to recharge, finding comfort in predictability and minimal external stimuli. However, his ADHD creates a constant craving for novelty, leading him to pursue new hobbies, social interactions and exciting activities like sports or spontaneous trips. This constant search for stimulation can lead to unfinished projects or shifting interests, meaning he abandons hobbies just as quickly as he picks them up.

This dynamic often results in cycles of stimulation followed by autistic burnout. James enjoys the thrill of new experiences, but they quickly drain his energy, requiring long periods of recovery in silence. To manage this, he carefully balances stimulating activities with periods of solitude, ensuring he has enough time to recover from the overstimulation that comes with his ADHD tendencies, while also meeting his autistic need for stability and predictability.

3. Structure vs Chaos

When I delivered my fifth TEDx talk on the theme *Order and Anarchy*, I was inspired by my father and others who navigate the intricate balance between structure and chaos. This duality of maintaining order amid inherent contradiction is a reflection of the lived experiences of many. When I was invited to speak at a twenty-four-hour global conference organised by ADHD UK, I decided to share this topic. Initially, the CEO expressed concern that the title *Order and Anarchy* might be perceived as offensive.

After discussing it with a patient focus group, they found that the concept deeply resonated with their experiences and perspectives, and embraced it enthusiastically.

Structure in Autism

In the realm of Autism, the concept of structure is multifaceted and deeply ingrained in the daily lives of individuals. Structure is not merely about organising physical spaces or adhering to routines; it embodies a comprehensive system that includes sequences, habits, planning and established algorithms for task completion. Each element within this system holds significant meaning and contributes to a sense of order and predictability.

For autistic individuals, structure might manifest in the way items are arranged – books could be systematically ordered by alphabetical criteria, genre or size. Habits and routines are followed with precise sequences, which are critical for maintaining a sense of control and stability. This meticulous attention to detail underscores that organisation is only a small component of the broader and more complex idea of structure.

When the established structure is disrupted – such as changes in task sequences, object placements or daily routine planning – it often leads to heightened anxiety and a sense of being overwhelmed. This disruption triggers an urgent need to re-establish order to regain a sense of normalcy and control. For autistic individuals, order and structure are not just preferences; they are foundational elements that constitute their second nature. These elements are deeply rooted values that provide a framework for understanding and interacting with the world.

The presence of structure brings a profound sense of happiness, joy and satisfaction. It ensures predictability, which is crucial for reducing anxiety and enhancing well-being. The intrinsic desire for structure is essential for their emotional and psychological stability. It allows them to navigate daily life with confidence and minimises the unpredictability that can lead to significant distress.

In essence, structure in Autism goes beyond the superficial aspects of tidiness and routine. It is a comprehensive system that supports the individual's need for predictability and control, ultimately fostering a sense of safety and contentment.

Chaos in ADHD

When one thinks of ADHD, the mind often conjures images of disorganisation, chaos, impulsivity and a relentless pursuit of activities that provide stimulation. Chaos in ADHD manifests as a perpetual state of unpredictability, deeply embedded in the core symptoms of inattention, hyperactivity and impulsivity. Individuals with ADHD frequently struggle to maintain focus, resulting in a fragmented approach to tasks and responsibilities. This can lead to unfinished projects, missed deadlines and a pervasive sense of disorganisation in daily life. The experience of chaos in ADHD is marked by carelessness, distraction and difficulty in completing tasks, all of which contribute to the disorder's complex and challenging nature.

Hyperactivity adds to this chaos by driving continuous movement and restlessness. The need for constant stimulation can cause individuals to jump from one activity to another without completing any, further amplifying the sense of chaos.

Impulsivity exacerbates the chaos, as individuals with ADHD often act without thinking, making spontaneous decisions that disrupt routines and plans. This impulsivity can manifest in behaviours such as interrupting conversations, making hasty purchases or engaging in risky activities without considering the consequences.

Together these symptoms create an environment where maintaining order and consistency is a significant challenge. Despite efforts to implement organisational strategies, the intrinsic characteristics of ADHD often make it difficult to sustain structure, leading to an ongoing cycle of chaos and attempts to restore control.

Structure and Chaos in AuDHD

In individuals with AuDHD, the coexistence of structure and chaos manifests in intriguing and often paradoxical ways. This duality is a hallmark of the unique interplay between Autism and ADHD, reflecting the complex nature of these co-occurring conditions.

You may find piles of clothes strewn across the floor, creating an impression of disorder and chaos in a person's living space. Yet amid this apparent disarray, you might discover a collection of figurines arranged with meticulous precision. Each item is perfectly aligned, reflecting an eye for detail and a deep appreciation for order. This juxtaposition of chaos and structure illustrates the multifaceted nature of AuDHD, where the need for organisation coexists with an underlying tendency towards disorder.

Individuals with AuDHD often embrace spontaneity, driven by a desire for novelty and excitement. However, they may simultaneously struggle with change, which can be unsettling due to the autistic preference for routine and predictability. This contradiction is mirrored in their approach to daily life: they thrive on routine yet may quickly become bored with repetitive tasks.

The alternating behaviours and inconsistencies in their actions are not merely quirks but essential aspects of their neurodivergent experience. These shifts reflect an ongoing negotiation between opposing tendencies as they navigate a world that requires both adaptability and consistency. This dynamic interplay creates a rich tapestry of experiences, offering insights into the nuanced and often contradictory nature of AuDHD.

> **Case Study 6:** Alex, a thirty-year-old architect with AuDHD, experiences a constant interplay between structure and chaos. At work, his autistic traits lead him to thrive in a highly organised and predictable environment. His workspace is meticulously arranged, and he follows a structured routine which provides him with a sense of control and stability. The precision and predictability of his job allow him to function at his best, ensuring projects are completed with attention to detail and care.
>
> In contrast, Alex's personal life is marked by the chaos driven by his ADHD. His apartment is often cluttered, with unfinished tasks and scattered belongings reflecting his difficulty maintaining order outside of work. Impulsivity and a need for novelty lead to spontaneous decisions and disorganised spaces, creating an ongoing struggle between the desire for routine and the disruptive effects of ADHD. This constant push-pull between structure and chaos defines Alex's experience, illustrating the complex and often contradictory nature of living with AuDHD.

4. Caution vs Risk-Taking

Caution in Autism

In the intricate world of Autism, caution and meticulousness play a central role in how individuals navigate their daily lives. Autism involves a heightened awareness of potential unpredictability and an inherent drive to avoid outcomes that provoke anxiety. This cautious approach means that autistic individuals often prefer to stick to familiar routines and environments, as the unknown can be a source of significant stress and discomfort.

For example, trying new activities or exploring uncharted territories can be daunting. The fear of unexpected results or unfamiliar sensory experiences can lead to a preference for predictability and routine. This cautiousness is not just about avoiding physical dangers but extends to social interactions and everyday choices. Autistic individuals may avoid engaging with strangers or new acquaintances, not because they lack interest, but because the unpredictability of these interactions can be overwhelming.

In social contexts, this caution can manifest as a tendency to remain quiet in meetings or social gatherings, especially when surrounded by unfamiliar faces. The complexity of interpreting social cues and the anxiety of miscommunication often result in a reserved demeanour. Autistic individuals might also avoid trying new routes or foods, as these changes introduce variables that disrupt their sense of stability and predictability.

However, this careful approach doesn't entirely shield them from challenging situations. Misreading social cues can sometimes lead to awkward moments, such as oversharing factual information with someone they perceive as trustworthy, even if that person is a stranger. These experiences highlight the delicate balance that autistic individuals maintain between protecting themselves from anxiety-inducing unpredictability and navigating the social world.

In essence, Autism is characterised by a deep-seated need for control and predictability. This need drives many of the behaviours and preferences observed in autistic individuals, from their careful social interactions to their steadfast routines. Understanding and respecting this need for caution can help to create supportive environments that accommodate their unique ways of engaging with the world.

Risk-Taking in ADHD

In the context of ADHD, risk-taking is not just a behaviour – it's a fundamental aspect of the condition. This drive for novelty and stimulation is rooted in the neurobiological need for dopamine, a neurotransmitter that plays a critical role in reward and pleasure pathways. Individuals with ADHD often seek out new experiences and take risks as a way to obtain the dopamine boosts their brains crave.

Engaging in risky behaviours provides a temporary increase in dopamine levels, which can help alleviate the chronic boredom and restlessness that many individuals with ADHD experience. This need for stimulation can manifest in a variety of ways, from pursuing adrenaline-pumping activities like extreme sports or thrill-seeking adventures, to more impulsive actions such as binge eating, compulsive shopping, or engaging in unsafe sexual behaviours.

For some, the quest for dopamine can lead to substance use, including drugs and alcohol, as these can provide the sought-after neurochemical rewards.

In my practice as a neurodevelopmental psychiatrist, I often draw on the wisdom of my mentor, who emphasised a crucial approach when discussing recreational substance use. He suggested a litmus test involving a specific enquiry about cocaine: asking individuals how it makes them feel. This question often reveals a paradoxical effect for many users. While cocaine is typically known for its stimulating properties, most individuals with ADHD report that it brings about a sense of clarity, focus, and a reduction in the mental busyness that often plagues their daily lives. This reaction, although not universal, is quite common and provides significant insights into an ADHD brain.

For most, the calming effect of cocaine can be indicative of their neurochemical profile and how their brain responds to stimulants. This response can be particularly telling for individuals with ADHD, as stimulants like cocaine and prescription medications such as methylphenidate (Ritalin) or amphetamine (Adderall) can have similar effects in terms of enhancing focus and reducing hyperactivity. Understanding this response helps clinicians to tailor their approach to treatment, ensuring that the interventions align with the individual's unique neurochemistry. This nuanced understanding of substance response underscores the importance of personalised medicine in the field of neurodevelopmental conditions. Unfortunately, this can sometimes result in legal troubles, as the impulsivity associated with ADHD might lead individuals to make decisions without fully considering the consequences.

Moreover, this relentless pursuit of new and exciting stimuli can interfere with the ability to focus on long-term goals and commitments. The constant need for change and the allure of the next novel experience often results in difficulty maintaining attention on more mundane or routine tasks. This can lead to a cycle of starting projects with great enthusiasm but struggling to see them through to completion.

The interplay between risk-taking and impulsivity in ADHD highlights the importance of understanding the underlying neurobiological mechanisms. Recognising this need for stimulation can guide more effective strategies for managing ADHD. For instance, finding healthy and structured ways to channel this need for novelty – such as engaging in creative hobbies, physical exercise or careers that provide variety and excitement – can help mitigate some of the more destructive behaviours associated with the condition.

AuDHD – Tug of War

In individuals with AuDHD there exists a dynamic interplay between caution and risk-taking, akin to a delicate tug of war. Autism, with its inherent need for predictability and safety, often acts as a tempering force, reining in the more anarchic tendencies of ADHD. It serves as a kind of internal parent, providing a stabilising influence that prevents impulsive risk-taking from leading to potentially dangerous outcomes.

Conversely, ADHD introduces an element of spontaneity and boldness into the mix, challenging the often overly cautious nature of Autism. This interaction fosters a balance where calculated risks can be taken – something that pure Autism might not easily permit. The impulsive drive of ADHD encourages ventures into new experiences and opportunities that, while carefully moderated by autistic caution, allow for growth and adaptability.

This symbiotic relationship ensures that the impulsivity of ADHD is kept in check, while the rigid caution of Autism is gently pushed towards embracing occasional risks. Together they create a unique equilibrium where both caution and risk-taking coexist, each tempering the excesses of the other and enabling a more balanced approach to navigating life's challenges. This interplay exemplifies the intricate dance between these two neurodivergent conditions, highlighting how they can complement each other in fostering a nuanced and adaptive behavioural repertoire.

> **Case Study 7:** Emily, a twenty-seven-year-old marketing specialist with AuDHD, experiences a constant tension between her autistic need for caution and predictability and her ADHD-driven impulse for risk-taking. At work, her Autism keeps her grounded, ensuring she follows routines meticulously and avoids unexpected changes. She prefers familiar, well-organised environments, which help her maintain a high level of performance. However, this cautiousness also limits her willingness to try new approaches, as she fears the unpredictability of unfamiliar strategies.
>
> Outside of work, her ADHD leads her to impulsive, thrill-seeking activities like spontaneous trips or extreme sports. These moments of risk-taking give her the excitement she craves, but her Autism often steps in to moderate her actions, preventing her

from making overly reckless decisions. This interplay between caution and impulsivity creates a balance in her life, where she can explore new experiences without losing the structure and stability that her autistic traits provide. Together, her Autism and ADHD form a unique equilibrium that allows her to navigate both routine and novelty in a way that fosters personal and professional growth.

5. Repetition vs Novelty

Repetition in Autism

In Autism, one of the hallmark diagnostic criteria is the tendency towards repetition. This repetition manifests in various aspects of daily life, reflecting a deep-seated preference for routine and familiarity. It includes repetitive pursuits of interests, consistent choices in daily activities, such as food and clothing, and even the enjoyment of watching the same movie multiple times. This penchant for repetition extends to travel preferences, where taking the same route, visiting the same destinations and staying in familiar accommodations become part of a comforting routine.

Repetition also plays a role in communication, with individuals often using the same words, phrases and metaphors in similar conversations. This repetitive pattern serves as a mechanism to avoid anxiety and steer clear of unfamiliar experiences or interactions with new people. However, once a new situation becomes familiar and understood, it can seamlessly integrate into the existing cycle of repetition.

For individuals with Autism, repetition is not a source of boredom but rather a source of comfort and stability.

They might happily watch the same movie over 200 times, read the same book repeatedly or maintain the same room decor for years. Similarly, taking the same route to work and back home provides a sense of predictability, and disruptions like roadworks requiring an alternative route can lead to frustration and anxiety.

Ultimately, repetition in Autism is not merely a rigid habit but a way to create a predictable and manageable world. It allows individuals to navigate life with a sense of control and reduces the anxiety associated with change and uncertainty. By understanding this aspect of Autism, caregivers and educators can create supportive environments that respect and accommodate the need for repetition while gently encouraging exploration and adaptation to new experiences.

Autism does not like novelty unless it's planned.

Novelty in ADHD

The ADHD brain thrives on a constant influx of stimulation. This is due to the neurological need for increased levels of dopamine and norepinephrine, which are chemicals that help regulate mood, attention and behaviour. The drive for novelty acts as a catalyst in releasing these neurotransmitters, making new and stimulating experiences particularly rewarding.

For individuals with ADHD, novelty can come in many forms. It might manifest as an exciting new project, starting a new job or immersing oneself in a hobby. The thrill of meeting new people, exploring unfamiliar places and forming new friendships also serves this need. Additionally, engaging in daredevil activities or acquiring new possessions can provide the excitement that the ADHD brain craves. It's important to note that what is stimulating for someone with ADHD may not necessarily be perceived the same way by others. This unique pursuit of excitement underscores the diversity in how people with ADHD experience and interact with the world around them.

An ADHD brain detests repetition.

Novelty and Repetition in AuDHD

In individuals with AuDHD, the coexistence of repetition and novelty is a fascinating phenomenon. On one hand, there is a profound need for new experiences, spontaneity and the occasional 'dopamine shot' that comes from engaging in novel activities. This drive can manifest in the pursuit of exciting adventures, new hobbies or meeting new people. Such pursuits provide the stimulation their brains crave, yet this constant need for novelty can sometimes make it challenging to maintain long-term jobs or relationships.

Conversely, people with AuDHD often find comfort in repetition and routine in certain aspects of their lives. They may exhibit a strong preference for sameness, whether it's eating the same foods, watching the same films or series, or consistently interacting with the same people. This paradoxical nature can lead to confusion as they navigate life, often harbouring the misconception that everyone shares these seemingly opposing tendencies. This duality can result in a lifelong struggle to understand and reconcile these contrasting needs, highlighting the complex interplay between the desire for stability and the craving for excitement that characterises the AuDHD experience.

In the intricate landscape of AuDHD, distinguishing between the behaviours attributed to ADHD and those associated with Autism can be remarkably challenging. This complexity often arises from the conflicting nature of their tendencies and mindset. Individuals with AuDHD may exhibit a blend of characteristics from both conditions, making it difficult for even seasoned professionals to pinpoint whether a particular behaviour stems from ADHD's impulsivity and need for novelty or Autism's preference for routine and repetition.

As a result, many individuals with AuDHD find themselves slipping through the diagnostic net. The overlapping and seemingly contradictory traits can obscure a clear understanding of their unique neurodevelopment profile. This ambiguity often leads to a lack of appropriate support and intervention, as the dual presence of ADHD and Autism creates a nuanced behavioural tapestry that can defy traditional diagnostic categories. Recognising and addressing this divergence is crucial for providing tailored care and understanding for those navigating the complexities of AuDHD.

> **Case Study 8:** Sam, a thirty-two-year-old IT specialist with AuDHD, experiences a constant internal struggle between his autistic need for repetition, like watching the same movie at least a hundred times, and his ADHD-driven craving for novelty. At work, Sam finds comfort in familiar routines. He takes the same route to the office daily, eats the same lunch and prefers to stick to familiar tasks that he can do without much unpredictability. This repetition helps him to stay grounded and reduces anxiety, providing a sense of

stability in his professional life. Even socially, Sam prefers interacting with a small, consistent group of people, finding comfort in the predictability of these interactions.

However, his ADHD traits introduce a craving for novelty that disrupts his carefully built routines. Sam often finds himself suddenly abandoning tasks or projects at work when something new and exciting captures his attention. In his personal life, he impulsively takes up new hobbies – like skydiving or learning an instrument – only to drop them quickly once the initial thrill fades. This push-pull between the need for routine and the desire for new experiences creates a constant tension in his life, leaving Sam struggling to find a balance between comfort and excitement, repetition and novelty.

6. Planning vs Spontaneity

Planning in Autism

Autism is often characterised by a preference for planning and structure, where routines, sequences and processes are meticulously followed. In this context, there is little tolerance for inconsistencies or deviations from established patterns. Life unfolds according to a carefully constructed algorithm, leaving no room for norm-defying insurgency.

This structured approach extends to both work and home environments. Daily tasks, such as errands, must be completed in a specific order, such as brushing teeth followed by taking a shower. Similarly, getting dressed requires adhering to a precise sequence, like putting on a shirt before pants and socks, with no deviations permitted. Books and clothes are arranged in a particular order, and any disruption can lead to a feeling of unease or an off day.

For those with Autism, last-minute changes or spontaneous plans can be unsettling. Holidays and excursions are planned well in advance, often with tickets booked six months to a year ahead. The itineraries are thoroughly prepared, with street views, parking spots and toilets meticulously marked on the map. Spontaneity is not their preference; instead, they find comfort in knowing that every detail is accounted for, allowing them to navigate their world with confidence and predictability.

Spontaneity in ADHD

In individuals with ADHD, boredom is a significant challenge, often making it difficult to sustain interest in a single hobby or activity. This restlessness stems from an inherent need for novelty, which helps to stimulate the production of dopamine and norepinephrine – neurotransmitters essential for motivation and pleasure.

Spontaneity is a defining characteristic of ADHD, manifesting as a preference for impulsive actions and a strong attraction to new and exciting experiences. The ADHD brain craves increased stimulation, and this desire drives the frequent release of dopamine. Consequently, individuals with ADHD often make rapid decisions without fully considering potential consequences, which can lead to unexpected adventures or risks. This impulsivity might involve spontaneous trips and purchases, or sudden changes in plans.

The search for novelty is a hallmark of the ADHD experience. New foods, activities or social connections provide the excitement and engagement that the ADHD brain seeks. With a low tolerance for routine and repetition, those with ADHD quickly become bored and are driven to seek new stimuli to maintain their interest.

Adaptability is another key trait, as people with ADHD are often able to switch gears effortlessly when plans change. They thrive in environments that embrace unpredictability, such as fast-paced jobs or dynamic social settings. Spontaneity in ADHD is typically accompanied by bursts of energy and enthusiasm, which can be channelled into creative projects or adventurous activities. When something captivates their interest, individuals with ADHD can immerse themselves fully, exploring it with intense focus before moving on just as quickly.

Social interactions are often spontaneous, with individuals suddenly deciding to meet friends or attend social gatherings without prior planning. This spontaneity can make them engaging and charismatic, drawing others to their dynamic personalities. However, while spontaneity offers excitement, it can also present challenges in maintaining long-term commitments and consistency in both personal and professional realms.

Despite these challenges, the ability to think outside the box is a notable strength of those with ADHD. Their spontaneous approach to problem-solving often leads to creative and innovative solutions. A willingness to experiment with new methods can result in significant achievements, particularly in fields that value creativity and innovation.

Planning vs Spontaneity in AuDHD

In individuals with AuDHD, there is a fascinating and dynamic interplay between planning and spontaneity, akin to a constant seesawing between these opposing forces. This unique balance is a testament to the complex interaction between Autism and ADHD, which shapes their behaviour and outlook in intriguing ways.

On one side of the spectrum, there is a strong resistance to change. This resistance is rooted in the autistic preference for structure and predictability. Individuals with AuDHD often find comfort and security in routines, which provide a sense of order and control in an otherwise unpredictable world. They may meticulously plan their daily activities, adhering to established schedules that help them navigate their day with confidence.

Yet, simultaneously, there exists a natural inclination towards spontaneity, driven by the ADHD component. This inclination brings with it an excitement for novelty and an eagerness to explore new experiences. While they may have carefully crafted plans, they are also capable of impulsive and unexpected actions that add a layer of unpredictability to their lives. This spontaneity can manifest in various ways, from whirlwind adventures to sudden changes in interests or hobbies.

The duality of structured routines and impulsive actions creates a unique and complex tapestry of behaviour in individuals with AuDHD. They are constantly balancing their need for stability with their desire for change, navigating a world where both elements are essential. This dynamic interplay requires them to be adaptable and resilient, as they find ways to harmonise these opposing forces in their daily lives.

> **Case Study 9:** Rachel, a twenty-eight-year-old project manager with AuDHD, struggles with the tension between her need for planning and her desire

for spontaneity. In her daily life, she relies heavily on routines – she plans her meals a week in advance, follows a strict morning routine and organises every aspect of her work with colour-coded calendars. She even prepares for social events well ahead of time, checking out the location online and mapping out her route. This meticulous planning helps Rachel to feel calm and in control.

Despite this, Rachel's ADHD often drives her to make impulsive decisions. On a whim, she might decide to rearrange her entire living room late at night, or she might buy tickets for a concert happening that same evening without any prior thought. She's also prone to spontaneous shopping sprees or trying out new hobbies, like learning to play the guitar, only to lose interest shortly after. These bursts of spontaneity give her the excitement she craves but clash with her need for predictability, leaving her to constantly navigate between her structured plans and sudden, impulsive actions.

7. Rigidity vs Change

Rigidity in Autism

Rigidity in Autism is characterised by a strong preference for routines, sameness and predictability. This tendency manifests in various ways and impacts multiple aspects of daily life, which we're now going to explore.

Individuals with Autism often thrive on routines and may have specific rituals for daily activities, such as morning routines or mealtimes. Any deviation from these can cause significant distress or anxiety. A structured environment provides a sense of security and comfort, while changes, such as rearranging furniture or altering a daily schedule, can be unsettling.

Resistance to change is a common feature in Autism. Transitions, whether between activities or during significant life changes like starting a new school or job, can be particularly challenging. New experiences or unfamiliar situations may feel overwhelming, leading individuals to prefer familiar activities, places and people.

Those with Autism often adhere rigidly to rules and expect others to do the same. This strict rule-following can lead to frustration when others do not meet the same standards. In play settings, they may favour games or activities with clear rules and struggle with imaginative play that lacks structure.

A preference for consistent sensory input, such as specific textures, sounds or lighting conditions, is another aspect of rigidity in Autism. Changes in sensory environments can cause discomfort or distress, further emphasising the need for predictability.

Rigidity can lead to heightened anxiety when faced with unexpected changes or disruptions. Emotional responses can be intense and may require support to manage. Uncertainty or ambiguous situations can be particularly challenging, as they lack the clear structure that individuals with Autism often rely on for comfort and understanding.

Change in ADHD

For individuals with ADHD, change is often a double-edged sword, serving as both a source of excitement and a potential challenge. The ADHD brain is inherently wired for novelty and stimulation, making the prospect of change particularly enticing. However, the accompanying impulsivity and difficulties with executive function can make adapting to change more complex.

Those with ADHD are frequently drawn to new and exciting experiences. Change offers the opportunity to explore fresh ideas, environments and activities, which can be exhilarating. This craving for novelty often leads to spontaneous decisions and a willingness to embrace the unknown. The prospect of something different is highly motivating, providing the stimulation on which the ADHD brain thrives.

The impulsivity in ADHD allows individuals to rapidly adapt to change, as they are often willing to dive head first into new situations without overthinking the consequences. While change can be thrilling, the ability to plan and organise effectively can be a challenge, making transitions potentially chaotic if not managed carefully, which seems to happen a lot in ADHD.

Consistency can be difficult for individuals with ADHD, as maintaining a routine may feel restrictive. Change can provide relief from the monotony of routine, yet it can also disrupt necessary structures that help to manage daily life. The frequent attraction to change can lead to difficulties in establishing and maintaining long-term habits or commitments.

Change evokes a range of emotions, from excitement about new possibilities to anxiety about the unknown. The anticipation of change may be thrilling, but the unpredictability can also be stressful. Sudden or unexpected changes in the environment or schedule can be particularly challenging, triggering emotional responses that may be difficult to manage.

Despite these challenges, people with ADHD often display remarkable adaptability, quickly adjusting to new circumstances and thinking on their feet. This flexibility is a significant strength, allowing them to thrive in dynamic environments, particularly in last-minute or crisis situations. The ability to embrace change with enthusiasm and resilience underscores the complex and multifaceted nature of ADHD, highlighting both the opportunities and challenges it presents.

Rigidity and Adaptability in AuDHD

I often wondered how a person could be both rigid and flexible at the same time. In my own experience, I found myself rigid when it came to adhering to sequences, honouring commitments, and distinguishing between right and wrong. Yet I was surprisingly flexible when making spontaneous decisions about meeting friends, going out or tackling challenging situations.

Despite my willingness to pursue spontaneity, I initially felt apprehensive. Once I overcame that initial hesitation, however, I often found excitement in these unplanned ventures. Reflecting on the activities I engaged in, I realised they still aligned with my core values and were far from anarchic. My impulsivity and spontaneity, while seemingly random, were guided by an internal compass that ensured they remained within the bounds of my value system. This realisation helped me understand that my flexibility was indeed measured and not as contradictory as it initially appeared. This is how it presents in AuDHD.

Case Study 10: Michelle, a thirty-five-year-old software developer with AuDHD, experiences a constant push and pull between rigidity and spontaneity in both her work and personal life. At work, Michelle is highly structured and methodical. She follows strict routines, plans her projects meticulously and completes tasks in a specific, organised sequence. Any sudden changes, such as last-minute project updates or impromptu meetings, can cause her significant stress and anxiety, as she values predictability and control. However, her ADHD-driven side occasionally compels her to take on new tasks or try unconventional approaches, injecting bursts of spontaneity and creativity into her work, sometimes at the expense of her carefully maintained structure.

In her personal life, Michelle also follows a set routine, preparing her meals at specific times and organising her home with precision. Yet her ADHD often pulls her towards spontaneous decisions – she might suddenly decide to rearrange her home furniture late at night or impulsively plan a last-minute weekend getaway. While these spontaneous actions bring excitement and variety into her life, they can disrupt her carefully organised environment, leading to temporary chaos. Michelle constantly navigates the balance between her autistic need for routine and her ADHD-driven desire for novelty, with rigidity providing stability, and spontaneity offering moments of excitement in both her work and personal life.

8. Solitary vs Crowd

Solitary Activities in Autism

For individuals on the Autism spectrum, solitary activities are not merely pastimes but profound avenues for self-discovery and inner tranquillity. These activities provide a sanctuary where the external world's cacophony and noises fade into the background, allowing for a deep and meditative focus. Whether through the stroke of a brush, the curl of a written word or the assembly of a puzzle, engaging in these solitary pursuits is a journey into the self, where the mind finds both joy and peace.

These activities serve as a bulwark against the unpredictability and chaos of the external world. They provide structure and predictability, which are like the steady hands of a comforting friend for those with Autism. By adhering to familiar routines and rituals, individuals can explore their interests in a controlled environment, navigating their passions and curiosities at their own rhythm and pace.

Moreover, solitary activities are profound channels for emotional and creative expression. In the quiet solitude of their own space, individuals on the spectrum can give voice to their inner thoughts and feelings through various media such as art, music or writing. These expressions are not bound by the conventions of social communication and offer a pure, unfiltered outlet for creativity and emotion.

Solitary pursuits also function as essential tools for emotional regulation. They act as a retreat, a place of refuge from the sensory overload and social demands that often characterise the everyday environments of those with Autism. Here, in the solitude of their own company, there is a profound peace – a stillness that can soothe the tumult of the outer world.

Finally, these activities cultivate independence and autonomy, empowering individuals with Autism to take charge of their lives. They build skills and confidence, fostering a sense of agency that transcends the activities themselves and influences broader aspects of life. Through solitary pursuits, individuals with Autism not only engage with the world on their own terms but also sculpt a self-identity that is anchored in self-assuredness and control.

Thus, solitary activities are far more than simple diversions for those with Autism – they are essential practices of self-care and personal growth, enabling a deeper connection with oneself and crafting a space of calm and creativity in a world that often moves too fast.

Crowding in ADHD

Crowding in individuals with ADHD involves feeling overwhelmed by too much going on around them or too many thoughts at once, which can greatly affect their ability to think and function effectively. Here's how crowding impacts those with ADHD.

Physical crowding: people with ADHD often struggle in environments that are very busy, like crowded public areas, cluttered rooms or active workplaces. These settings can create sensory overload, bombarding the brain with too much visual and auditory information to process efficiently. In such crowded places, the overload of people, noise and activity can increase stress and anxiety, making it hard to focus and causing irritation, restlessness and discomfort. Handling these environments also demands spatial and situational awareness, which can be challenging for those with difficulties in attention and executive function.

Mental crowding: on the mental side, crowding occurs when someone with ADHD has too many thoughts, ideas or emotional responses vying for attention simultaneously. This can feel like a constantly racing mind that never pauses. This type of crowding can be as overwhelming as physical crowding and is a common issue for those with ADHD. It often results in trouble focusing on a single task, making decisions or organising thoughts clearly.

Additionally, mental crowding can trigger intense emotional reactions to ordinary situations, which might seem manageable to others. Difficulty in filtering out unnecessary emotional input can cause sudden mood swings or exaggerated responses to daily stresses. Initially, insomnia could be an outcome of a busy mind.

Solitude and Crowding in AuDHD

In the intricate interplay of Autism and ADHD, individuals often exhibit a nuanced balance between the desire for social interaction and the need for solitude. While there is an inherent wish to engage socially, there is also a strong inclination to retreat into solitude after a certain point, using this 'me time' to replenish depleted energy. The preference for one's own company and the solitude that accompanies it are neither extreme nor isolating; instead, they reflect a vital self-care practice that maintains emotional and mental balance.

This dynamic can oscillate, much like a seesaw, between periods of social engagement and solitude. Such shifts may be influenced by physical exertion, which has a notable effect on the often-racing minds characteristic of those with AuDHD. Engaging in physical activity helps to dissipate excess energy, which in turn can quiet the mind and lead to improved sleep patterns – a crucial element for overall well-being.

In the context of AuDHD, the oscillation between solitude and social engagement can sometimes result in one or both needs being overlooked. Individuals may struggle to find a sustainable rhythm, occasionally missing the cues that signify a need for rest or interaction. Recognising and respecting these alternating needs is crucial for managing AuDHD effectively, ensuring that individuals can navigate their environments in a way that honours their unique neurodivergent needs.

> **Case Study 11:** Sophie, a forty-year-old astrophysicist with AuDHD, manages a delicate balance between her need for solitude and the demands of a busy family life, alongside her ADHD-driven desire for social engagement. At work, Sophie prefers quiet and uninterrupted time to focus on her research, finding deep satisfaction in solitary activities like analysing data or writing papers. This solitude allows her to immerse herself in complex theories, providing a controlled and predictable environment where she can thrive intellectually without the distractions of social interaction, which her Autism often makes overwhelming.
>
> However, Sophie's ADHD pulls her towards spontaneous social interactions, both at work and at home. She enjoys collaborative discussions with her colleagues, and occasionally seeks out conferences and networking opportunities for the stimulation and excitement they bring. At home, as a married mother, Sophie often dives into family activities with enthusiasm, juggling the social demands of raising children and managing household duties. However, after extended periods of busy family life or work gatherings, Sophie feels drained and retreats to moments of solitude to recharge. This constant

oscillation, between engaging with her children and work colleagues while needing alone time, creates a challenging but necessary balance for her well-being, as she navigates the interplay between solitude and crowding in both her professional and personal life.

Is AuDHD a New Diagnosis?

The term AuDHD represents a colloquial blend of Autism and Attention Deficit Hyperactivity Disorder (ADHD) used to describe individuals who exhibit characteristics of both conditions.

This designation has gained traction within both clinical practice and everyday language as a way to encapsulate the complex interplay of symptoms that do not entirely fit within the traditional frameworks of either disorder/condition alone. However, it is important to note that AuDHD is not officially recognised as a distinct diagnosis within the major diagnostic manuals, such as the *Diagnostic and Statistical Manual of Mental Disorders, Fifth Edition* (DSM-5) or the *International Classification of Diseases* (ICD-11).

Understanding AuDHD

The convergence of symptoms in individuals displaying traits of both Autism and ADHD presents unique clinical challenges and has implications for treatment. Autism is characterised by difficulties in social interaction, fixed interests and repetitive behaviours, and challenges with communication. ADHD is marked by patterns of inattention, hyperactivity and impulsivity. When these symptoms overlap, they can compound or alter the manifestation/presentation of each other, creating a clinical picture that might not be fully addressed by interventions typically used for either condition alone.

Clinical Implications

The discussion of AuDHD in clinical settings underscores a critical need for personalised treatment plans that address a wider array of symptoms. Traditional ADHD treatments focusing on improving attention and reducing hyperactivity might not suffice if an individual also needs support in social communication and managing sensory sensitivities common in Autism. It is observed that when the ADHD aspect of AuDHD is addressed through treatment, the characteristics of Autism often become more noticeable. This change in prominence can lead some to mistakenly believe that medications used to manage ADHD might cause Autism. However, this is a misconception. The treatment merely reduces the symptoms of ADHD, which can make the traits associated with Autism more apparent, but it does not induce or exacerbate Autism itself.

Diagnostic Challenges

One of the main challenges with the concept of AuDHD is the risk of oversimplification or misdiagnosis. A careful and thorough evaluation is essential to accurately attribute each symptom to its correct source and to ensure that the needs associated with both Autism and ADHD are fully addressed. This requires a deep and comprehensive understanding of both conditions, along with an in-depth knowledge of their respective diagnostic criteria. Moreover, it is crucial to recognise the overlapping symptoms of Autism and ADHD and to be sensitive to the ways these conditions interact, considering cultural, religious and social nuances.

For a neurodevelopmental psychiatrist, being well-versed in both Autism and ADHD is imperative for accurately diagnosing AuDHD. This expertise makes it possible to discern subtle distinctions and ensure that each individual's unique presentation is understood and treated appropriately, thereby optimising care and support.

Research and Future Directions

Research into the co-occurrence of ASD and ADHD is still evolving. Studies have begun to explore the genetic, neurobiological and environmental factors that might contribute to their overlap. Understanding these connections is crucial for developing more effective diagnostic tools and treatments. Both these conditions involve frontal lobe and executive functions.

The ongoing discussion about AuDHD reflects a broader movement within the field of neurodevelopmental conditions towards recognising the fluidity of diagnostic categories. This perspective advocates for a spectrum-based approach rather than strict categorical diagnoses, suggesting that neurodevelopmental conditions can exhibit a broad range of overlapping symptoms that need to be managed with a flexible, personalised approach.

Why a Sudden Rise in AuDHD?

Until 2013, the official diagnostic criteria did not permit a dual diagnosis of Autism Spectrum Condition (ASC) and Attention Deficit Hyperactivity Condition (ADHD) within the same individual. However, clinicians and researchers had long observed the coexistence of these conditions. The term 'official' is pivotal here, as it marks a turning point where what was previously an informal understanding among experts became recognised in diagnostic manuals. Prior to this acknowledgment many cases of ADHD in individuals with Autism were indirectly attributed to mere hyperactivity or inattention and managed accordingly with stimulants.

The formal recognition in 2013 that ASD and ADHD can co-occur has significant implications. It suggests that there may be a substantial backlog of cases from past decades – a backlog compounded by previous diagnostic frameworks that did not accommodate the complex interplay between these conditions. If we accept current estimates suggesting a co-occurrence rate of 50–70 per cent for AuDHD, it becomes clear that, historically, many individuals may have been either undiagnosed or misdiagnosed. This has left numerous people without proper management for their conditions, leading them to prolonged searches for identity and answers, hence the looming waiting lists.

The rise in visibility and diagnosis of AuDHD in recent years is often simplistically attributed to phenomena such as the pandemic and the pervasive influence of social media. While these factors have undoubtedly played a role in shaping public awareness and discourse, they overshadow more critical underlying issues. Key among these is the insufficient training and preparedness of healthcare professionals to recognise and treat the nuanced interaction of Autism and ADHD. Despite the high prevalence of these co-occurring conditions, there has been a global shortfall in developing the necessary skills among healthcare workers to meet the needs of this group.

Instead of acknowledging these gaps and the resulting challenges they pose, there is a tendency to blame external factors like social media or pandemic-related disruptions. This misattribution does a disservice to those affected, diverting attention from the urgent need to enhance professional training, expand services and improve diagnostic criteria to better reflect the realities of neurodevelopmental diversity. As we move forward, it is crucial that we address these shortcomings to provide more comprehensive and effective support for individuals with AuDHD.

How to Spot AuDHD?

AuDHD may not present as pure Autism or pure ADHD in a person. Hence, it's necessary to look beyond the obvious, exploring the nuances of each. Clinicians need to be more observant, be more enthusiastic listeners and have greater in-depth knowledge of the subject.

I recall a pivotal moment during a consultation that highlighted the importance of careful communication and observation when assessing neurodevelopmental conditions. While speaking with a patient, I posed what I thought was a straightforward question: 'Who's the eldest of the lot?' This was meant as a follow-up to an earlier enquiry about siblings. The patient replied with sincerity and precision, 'Of course, my parents. My dad is the eldest, followed by my mum, then my sister, me, and finally my brother.'

This literal interpretation of my question was a telling moment. I had intended to ask, 'Who's the eldest among you siblings?' but my phrasing inadvertently prompted a more comprehensive answer. The patient's response illuminated a detail that might otherwise have been overlooked. Their literal interpretation of language hinted at characteristics often associated with Autism, such as a preference for precision and concrete thinking over implied or abstract meanings.

This exchange encouraged me to delve deeper into the possibility of Autism, guiding the subsequent evaluation and ultimately leading to a diagnosis. It was a reminder of the subtle cues that can reveal underlying neurodevelopmental differences, underscoring the significance of clear communication and attentive listening in clinical practice. This experience reinforced the notion that every interaction holds the potential to uncover crucial insights, shaping our understanding and approach to each unique individual.

The underlying features of conditions like Autism and ADHD can manifest in various nuanced ways, such as a literal thought process, distinct types of interactions, or a tendency to disengage from conversations. Individuals may also experience sensory overload, display resistance to change or structured environments, and exhibit a preoccupation with specific interests. It is crucial to remain vigilant in identifying these subtle characteristics, as they often require careful observation and understanding. Recognising these nuances is essential for providing appropriate support and fostering an environment that accommodates and respects individual differences.

Diagnosing AuDHD involves a multidisciplinary approach, typically engaging psychologists, psychiatrists and other professionals. This process includes clinical interviews with caregivers to discuss developmental history, behaviour patterns and family history, as well as observational assessments to evaluate how individuals interact in various settings. Standardised tests may also be used to assess cognitive functions, attention, social understanding and emotional regulation; however, there has not been a standardised measure developed to diagnose both Autism and ADHD together.

Identifying AuDHD can be challenging due to overlapping symptoms, making it difficult to distinguish behaviours attributed to Autism from those of ADHD. For example, a child's difficulty with change might be interpreted as ADHD impulsivity. Hence, the professional needs to be extremely well versed in both Autism and ADHD, understanding their nuances, variations, cultural sensitivities and manifestations.

A comprehensive evaluation of both ASD and ADHD symptoms is crucial, considering the individual's overall functioning across different environments. Professionals must understand how the coexistence of these conditions uniquely shapes an individual's experiences and behaviours. As understanding of AuDHD grows, diagnostic approaches and interventions will continue to evolve, aiming to provide better support for people with this dual diagnosis.

Why and How Is AuDHD missed?

The co-occurrence of Autism and Attention Deficit Hyperactivity Disorder (ADHD) is frequently missed or misdiagnosed for several reasons, including the complexity of overlapping symptoms, diagnostic challenges and lack of awareness. Here are some key factors that explain why AuDHD is often overlooked.

Overlapping Symptoms

1. **Shared characteristics:** Autism and ADHD share several symptoms, such as difficulties with attention, executive functioning and social interaction. These overlapping traits can make it challenging to distinguish between the two conditions.

2. **Masking effects:** the presence of one condition can mask the symptoms of the other. For example, the hyperactivity and impulsivity associated with ADHD may overshadow the social communication difficulties seen in Autism; likewise, Autism can mask the attentional difficulties in ADHD.

3. **Variability:** both ASD and ADHD present with a wide range of symptoms that vary in severity. This variability can make it difficult for clinicians to recognise the dual diagnosis, especially if the symptoms of one condition are more pronounced.

Diagnostic Challenges

1. **Historical diagnostic criteria:** until 2013, it was not officially recognised that a person could be diagnosed with both ASD and ADHD. As a result, many individuals who met the criteria for both conditions may have been diagnosed with only one or none.

2. **Inadequate screening tools:** many diagnostic tools are designed to assess either ASD or ADHD, but not both simultaneously. This can lead to partial assessments that miss the nuances of co-occurring symptoms.

3. **Focus on primary symptoms:** clinicians may focus on the most obvious or disruptive symptoms, often those associated with ADHD, and overlook the more subtle signs of Autism, particularly in individuals who have learned to mask their social difficulties.

Lack of Awareness and Training

1. **Limited professional training:** many healthcare providers lack training in recognising the co-occurrence of ASD and ADHD, leading to a narrow diagnostic focus. This can result in missed or misdiagnosed cases of AuDHD.

2. **Stereotypes and misconceptions:** there are persistent stereotypes about both Autism and ADHD that can obscure a dual diagnosis. For instance, the misconception that individuals with Autism cannot have high energy or that those with ADHD cannot have social communication difficulties may prevent clinicians from considering both conditions.

Social and Cultural Factors

1. **Gender differences:** AuDHD is often underdiagnosed in girls and women, largely due to gender-based stereotypes and the subtle differences in how symptoms manifest between genders. Unlike boys, who may display more overt hyperactivity, girls with AuDHD often present with less visible signs, such as internalised symptoms, that can easily be overlooked. These symptoms might include

anxiety, perfectionism or social withdrawal, which do not align with the traditional expectations of how ADHD presents. Consequently, these differences can result in a lack of recognition and understanding, leading to many girls and women not receiving the diagnosis and support they need. It is essential for clinicians to be aware of these gender-related nuances to ensure accurate diagnosis and to provide appropriate interventions for females with AuDHD.

2. **Cultural perceptions:** cultural norms and expectations significantly impact how symptoms of conditions like Autism and ADHD are perceived and reported, which can lead to underdiagnosis or misdiagnosis in certain populations. In some cultures, behaviours associated with these conditions may be interpreted differently, either minimising their visibility or attributing them to other causes. Furthermore, the support structures provided by family and society – often referred to as 'scaffolding' – can mask the presence of AuDHD until later stages of life. This support may help individuals to manage their symptoms to a degree, delaying the recognition and diagnosis of their condition. Understanding these cultural dynamics is essential for healthcare professionals to ensure accurate diagnosis and treatment across diverse populations.

Is AuDHD a TikTok Diagnosis?

With the advent of social media, there has been a noticeable shift in how mental health issues, such as AuDHD, are discussed and perceived. This shift has led to an increase in both referrals for professional evaluation and instances of self-diagnosis. As social media platforms continue to grow in influence, they have become both a source of information and misinformation, resulting in a complex dynamic regarding mental health awareness and diagnosis.

The Role of Social Media in Mental Health Awareness

1. **Increased visibility and awareness:** social media platforms like TikTok, Instagram and YouTube have made information about mental health conditions more accessible to a broader audience. Users share personal stories and experiences, helping to reduce stigma and increase awareness of conditions like ADHD. This greater visibility has encouraged more people to seek professional help and understand their symptoms.

2. **Community support and validation:** online communities provide a space for individuals to connect with others who share similar experiences. This sense of belonging and validation can be empowering for people who have felt misunderstood or isolated. Hearing others describe symptoms and coping strategies can prompt individuals to seek a professional diagnosis, increasing the number of referrals.

3. **Quick and accessible information:** social media offers bite-sized content that is easily digestible and widely shared. Short videos and posts can quickly

disseminate information about symptoms, treatment options and personal experiences, making mental health topics more approachable.

The Challenges of Social Media in Diagnosis

1. **Misinformation and oversimplification:** while social media can spread awareness, it can also propagate misinformation and oversimplify complex conditions like AuDHD. Users may present symptoms in a way that lacks nuance, leading to misunderstandings about the condition. This can result in people self-diagnosing based on incomplete or incorrect information.

2. **Trends and virality:** mental health topics can become trends on social media, leading to the spread of certain narratives or symptoms that gain popularity. As these narratives go viral, they can create pressure to identify with certain diagnoses, even if they are not accurate. This phenomenon can lead to an increase in self-diagnosis without professional consultation.

3. **Confirmation bias:** people may seek out content that confirms their suspicions about having a particular condition. Algorithms that tailor content to users' interests can exacerbate this by continually presenting similar material, thus reinforcing self-diagnosed beliefs without critical evaluation.

The Increase in Referrals and Self-Diagnosis

1. **Empowerment and advocacy:** for some, social media provides the knowledge and confidence

needed to seek professional evaluation, leading to a rise in referrals. Access to shared experiences can empower individuals to advocate for their health and seek a formal diagnosis. Self-diagnosis does not mean a formal diagnosis.

2. **Misdiagnosis and mismanagement:** on the flip side, self-diagnosis based on social media content can lead to misdiagnosis and mismanagement of mental health conditions. Without professional assessment, individuals may pursue inappropriate treatments or misunderstand their own experiences.

3. **The responsibility of content creators and platforms:** as social media continues to influence mental health awareness, content creators and platforms have a responsibility to ensure that information is accurate and balanced. This includes promoting content from reputable sources and encouraging users to seek professional advice for diagnosis and treatment.

Process of Learning through Generations

I believe that each generation has developed its own distinct ways of acquiring knowledge and navigating life. Baby Boomers grew up in an era where encyclopaedias and newspapers were the primary sources of information, providing a foundation for lifelong learning. For Generation X, television became a powerful medium, offering educational programming and documentaries that expanded their understanding of the world.

With the rise of the internet, Millennials had unprecedented access to information at their fingertips, allowing them to explore diverse topics and perspectives through online articles, forums and videos. Today, Generation Z and the emerging Generation Alpha are immersed in digital landscapes, where social media Reels and AI-driven platforms shape their learning experiences. TikTok, Instagram and YouTube offer bite-sized content, making information more accessible but also more susceptible to oversimplification and error.

In this age of information abundance, we face the dual challenge of navigating both knowledge and disinformation. It is our responsibility to critically evaluate the content we encounter, ensuring that we separate credible sources from those that are questionable. This is especially important for complex topics like AuDHD, which can easily become entangled in misconceptions. For example, dismissing AuDHD as merely a 'TikTok diagnosis' undermines the genuine experiences of individuals who live with the condition, and can lead to misinformation about its causes, symptoms and treatments.

To prevent such misunderstandings, we must foster media literacy and encourage critical thinking. This means questioning the validity of sources, cross-referencing information and engaging in thoughtful discussions. By doing so, we can help to ensure that the narrative around AuDHD and other important topics remains accurate, empowering individuals to make well-informed decisions and advocate for themselves and others in an increasingly complex world.

Chapter 6: Is AuDHD a Separate Diagnosis?

For as long as I can remember, I've lived with a constant, conflicting tension between my brain's relentless drive for order and my equally relentless inability to organise. I've always felt like I've had one foot in two different worlds: one that craved structure and focus, and another that seemed determined to scatter my attention in every direction. As a child, I never understood why I couldn't bring these two worlds together – why I felt like I was chasing my own mind, unable to pin it down long enough to do what was asked of me.

In retrospect, I now know that I was living with AuDHD, but at the time, I just felt like I was falling short. I struggled with focus and order, often feeling trapped in the space between needing to organise my world and being utterly unable to do so. It was a constant battle, one that I fought on my own without knowing there were others like me.

The Challenge of Hyperfocus and Inattention

Looking back, one of the most defining moments of my academic life was preparing for my paediatric written exam. It was the night before the test, and I hadn't even begun to review the curriculum. With panic setting in, my brain switched into its default state of hyperfocus. I stayed up all night, diving into textbooks and reviewing materials at a speed that should have been impossible; yet somehow, thanks to this hyperfocus, I made it through the entire curriculum without sleeping a wink. The next day, despite the exhaustion, I aced the exam, even earning a merit.

It was a baffling experience, one that left me both proud and deeply confused. How could I manage to pull off something so monumental in such a short period of time? And yet, despite this last-minute victory, I knew something wasn't right. It wasn't sustainable, and it certainly wasn't healthy.

The irony of my academic life was that while I could hyperfocus under pressure, there were other subjects – like ENT (ear, nose and throat) – that I loved so much and studied extensively, reading three reference books and teaching my friends. I became something of an expert among my peers, yet when it came time to take the exam, I barely managed to score well. I knew the material inside and out, but my brain couldn't focus in the exam hall. I couldn't sit still long enough or became too distracted to apply the knowledge I'd worked so hard to accumulate. My experience with ENT was a perfect example of how my brain worked against me, giving me the gift of deep knowledge but taking away my ability to perform when it mattered most.

Childhood Fascinations and Frustrations

My childhood was filled with moments that now, in hindsight, make perfect sense. As a young boy, I was completely obsessed with fast cars and motorcycles. I collected over 300 miniature vehicles and spent hours watching the world outside my school, counting how many Suzukis, Yamahas, Kawasakis and Hondas drove by. These were the moments I could lose myself in, being deeply focused and completely captivated by the subject matter.

But that same child who could count motorcycles for hours was also the child who forgot his homework. I constantly lost my notebooks, left my school supplies scattered in the classroom and found myself on the receiving end of my teachers' frustration. My mother, bless her, often completed my notebooks for me because I would misplace them so frequently. It wasn't that I didn't care about schoolwork; I did. But my brain was wired differently, and that wiring made it impossible for me to hold on to details that seemed so easy for other children.

Navigating a Mind in Overdrive

There were other parts of my life where my dual diagnosis showed itself in ways I couldn't understand at the time. For example, I always had trouble getting to sleep. My brain would go into overdrive the moment I tried to rest. Thoughts would race through my mind, jumping from one subject to another, making it impossible to drift off. It felt like my brain never wanted to stop, even when my body was desperate for sleep.

I never could understand why I struggled to focus on linguistics, a subject that required sustained attention and detailed thinking, but could spend hours immersed in math or biology, learning complex concepts and solving problems. It was as if my brain was wired to embrace the things that stimulated it the most while rejecting anything that required a methodical, step-by-step approach.

Socialising: a Delicate Balance

Social interactions were another realm where I felt constantly out of step with the world. Meeting new people was exhausting for me. I didn't like it. But growing up in a culture that valued social interactions, I had no choice but to learn to socialise. I became good at masking my discomfort, learning how to engage with others even when I felt like retreating into myself. People thought I was a quiet person, but those who knew me well — my family and close friends — saw a different side of me. In their company I was talkative and could easily dominate a conversation.

Despite my ability to mask and my occasional bursts of social energy, I felt a profound sense of self-doubt. I didn't understand why I was the way I was, and it gnawed at me. For years my confidence was shattered and my self-esteem lay in pieces. Even when I achieved something significant, I found myself attributing it to coincidence rather than ability. I lived with the constant feeling that I wasn't good enough, that I was somehow fundamentally flawed.

The Moment of Clarity

It wasn't until I received my AuDHD diagnosis that the pieces of the puzzle began to fall into place. Suddenly, everything made sense — the hyperfocus, the inattention, the deep love for certain subjects combined with the inability to organise my thoughts when it mattered most. I came to realise that my father, too, had been living with AuDHD, though neither he nor anyone around him understood it at the time. Seeing my father through this new lens allowed me to better understand myself. It was as if the fog that had clouded my sense of self for so long had finally lifted, and I could see clearly.

Now I understand that my Autism is where I draw my perseverance and my grit. It's why I can immerse myself so fully in the things I care about, why I don't give up easily, and why I hold on to the things that matter to me. At the same time, my ADHD is where my creativity comes from – it's the source of my energy and my innovation, the reason why I'm always looking for new ways to solve problems or approach challenges.

Paying It Forward: My Role as an Advocate

Having come to understand my own AuDHD, I carry this knowledge into my work with others. I've made it my mission to advocate for those who live with Autism, ADHD and AuDHD, helping them to navigate the same challenges I once faced. I use my experiences to guide others, offering them the validation and support that I so desperately needed when I was younger.

Every individual with AuDHD is unique. As I often remind my patients, 'If you've seen one person with AuDHD, you've seen just one person with AuDHD.' No two stories are the same. But what unites us all is the common thread of complexity – the push and pull of two conditions that shape our lives in ways both challenging and beautiful.

The Rise of AuDHD

In recent years the co-occurrence of Autism Spectrum Condition (ASC) and Attention Deficit Hyperactivity Disorder (ADHD), colloquially termed AuDHD, has garnered significant attention in both clinical practice and research. This is not merely a coincidence of two common neurodevelopmental conditions existing side by side; instead, it highlights a deeper, more complex interaction between Autism and ADHD. As we begin to understand the shared neurobiological underpinnings and behavioural traits that define these conditions, the need to recognise and address AuDHD has become increasingly clear. This intersection represents a growing area of interest, leading many clinicians and researchers to question whether AuDHD should be considered its own distinct diagnosis, or a reflection of how various neurodevelopmental conditions can overlap and interact.

Autism and ADHD have traditionally been seen as separate diagnoses, each with its own set of symptoms and treatment strategies. Autism is often characterised by difficulties with social communication, restricted and repetitive behaviours, and sensory sensitivities, while ADHD typically presents with inattention, impulsivity and hyperactivity. However, clinical evidence now suggests that these conditions frequently co-occur, with up to more than 50 per cent of individuals diagnosed with Autism also meeting the criteria for ADHD, and a significant percentage of individuals with ADHD exhibiting traits of Autism. The more we learn about this overlap, the more it challenges our current understanding of these conditions as discrete, stand-alone diagnoses.

The growing recognition of AuDHD has sparked a new conversation: is AuDHD its own diagnosis, or is it part of a broader neurodevelopmental spectrum? This question is central to understanding how we should approach individuals who display features of both Autism and ADHD. If we see AuDHD as a distinct diagnosis, it could lead to a more targeted approach in both diagnosis and treatment. On the other hand, if we consider Autism and ADHD as part of a broader neurodevelopmental spectrum, AuDHD may simply represent a point where these two conditions intersect, rather than being a separate entity.

This chapter seeks to explore both sides of this debate. The goal is to offer a comprehensive understanding of AuDHD, not only as a concept but also as a clinical reality that affects individuals across their lifespan. Whether it is regarded as a distinct diagnosis or a part of the neurodevelopmental spectrum, AuDHD is shaping how we think about and address the needs of individuals who present with dual diagnoses.

Is AuDHD a Separate Diagnosis or Part of a Neurodevelopmental Spectrum?

One of the most compelling aspects of AuDHD is how it forces us to reconsider traditional diagnostic frameworks. The DSM-5 allows for the co-diagnosis of Autism and ADHD, but it treats them as distinct entities with separate diagnostic criteria. Autism, for example, is primarily diagnosed based on deficits in social communication and the presence of repetitive behaviours, while ADHD is diagnosed based on patterns of inattention, impulsivity and hyperactivity. These diagnostic categories, however, fail to capture the lived experience of individuals who exhibit features of both conditions simultaneously.

For many people with both Autism and ADHD, the experience of living with these conditions is not one of separation but rather one of constant interaction. ADHD's impulsivity and inattention can exacerbate Autism's social challenges, and Autism's preference for routine can conflict with ADHD's need for novelty and stimulation. The reality of living with AuDHD is far more complex than any diagnostic manual can capture.

This has led some clinicians and researchers to propose that Autism and ADHD may not be entirely separate conditions but instead represent different points on a broader neurodevelopmental spectrum. This view suggests that the brain differences that underlie Autism and ADHD share common roots, and that individuals may exhibit traits of both conditions depending on where they fall on this spectrum. From this perspective, AuDHD is not a new diagnosis but a recognition of the natural overlap between Autism and ADHD, and the fact that many individuals experience a blend of traits from both conditions.

However, others argue that AuDHD should be considered a distinct clinical entity, separate from either Autism or ADHD alone. The reasoning behind this view is that the interaction of Autism and ADHD creates a unique set of challenges that cannot be adequately addressed by treating each condition individually. For instance, someone with AuDHD might require different treatment strategies than someone with only Autism or only ADHD. Recognising AuDHD as its own diagnosis could lead to more personalised and effective treatment approaches that address the full range of difficulties experienced by individuals with both conditions.

The Increasing Clinical Importance of Dual Diagnoses Across the Lifespan

The recognition of AuDHD is not just a theoretical exercise – it has profound implications for clinical practice, particularly in terms of how we approach diagnosis and treatment across the lifespan. Historically, both Autism and ADHD were viewed primarily as childhood conditions, with diagnosis and treatment largely focused on children. However, we now know that these conditions persist into adulthood and often present differently in adults compared to children. This is especially true for individuals with dual diagnoses of Autism and ADHD.

In my practice I have seen how the dual diagnosis of Autism and ADHD can manifest in adults who may have gone undiagnosed or misdiagnosed for years. Many of these individuals present with a complex array of symptoms that are difficult to categorise using traditional diagnostic criteria. For example, an adult with AuDHD might struggle with maintaining attention at work, managing social relationships and dealing with sensory sensitivities – all while navigating the expectations of adulthood. These individuals often report feeling misunderstood or inadequately supported, as treatments designed for Autism might not address their ADHD symptoms, and vice versa.

The importance of recognising AuDHD across the lifespan cannot be overstated. Many adults with dual diagnoses report that their symptoms were overlooked in childhood, particularly if one condition was more prominent than the other. For example, an individual with strong social communication difficulties might have been diagnosed with Autism early on, while their ADHD symptoms went unnoticed. Conversely, a child diagnosed with ADHD might not have received an Autism diagnosis until much later, after years of struggling with sensory processing or social difficulties.

The waiting lists that we see now are a backlog of six decades of not understanding and spotting Autism and ADHD, and now AuDHD.

By acknowledging the dual diagnosis of AuDHD, we can better support individuals throughout their lives, providing treatments that address the unique interplay between Autism and ADHD, rather than treating each condition in isolation. This is particularly important in adults, who may have developed coping mechanisms to manage their symptoms but still face significant challenges in their personal and professional lives. For these individuals a dual diagnosis can be life-changing, offering a new perspective on their struggles and opening the door to more effective treatments.

My Experience with AuDHD

I have spent much of my career working with individuals of all ages who present with dual diagnoses of Autism and ADHD, and also lived with Autism and ADHD. I struggled in my earlier years with my attention and concentration, as lessons became more complex and my attention span dwindled. I have also dealt with being distracted and disorganised while still being someone who was fascinated by organisation. From a very young age I would list things, such as cricket stats, films or stamps; every interest of mine was organised and had a pattern to it.

I have seen first-hand how complex and nuanced these cases can be.

Early in my career, I became interested in how Autism and ADHD intersected, particularly in adults who had long gone without a full understanding of their condition. I noticed that many of my patients who had been diagnosed with one condition were exhibiting traits of the other, leading me to explore the possibility of dual diagnoses.

Over the years, my work with AuDHD has expanded to include both children and adults, and I have come to appreciate the unique challenges faced by individuals with both conditions. In children, AuDHD often presents as a mix of social difficulties, hyperactivity and inattention, which can make school and peer relationships particularly challenging.

In adults, AuDHD can manifest as difficulties with work, social interactions and sensory overload, often leading to feelings of frustration and isolation.

One of the most important lessons I have learned through my work with AuDHD is that no two individuals experience it the same way. Autism and ADHD interact differently in each person, creating a wide range of features and challenges. This is why a one-size-fits-all approach to diagnosis and treatment simply does not work. Instead, it is essential to take a holistic, individualised approach that considers the full range of an individual's neurodevelopmental profile.

I have also seen how transformative it can be for people to receive a dual diagnosis of Autism and ADHD. Many of my patients have expressed relief at finally understanding why they have struggled in certain areas of their lives, bursting into tears or becoming emotional. They appreciate the opportunity to receive more targeted treatments that address both conditions. For some, a dual diagnosis has provided a sense of validation and clarity that they have long been seeking.

The rise of AuDHD marks a new frontier in our understanding of neurodevelopmental conditions.

Whether it is ultimately recognised as a separate diagnosis or as part of a broader spectrum, the growing recognition of the co-occurrence of Autism and ADHD is changing how we think about and treat these conditions.

The Spectrum Debate: Is AuDHD a Spectrum?

When you work in the world of neurodevelopmental conditions, you quickly realise that the brain doesn't follow the neat boundaries we might wish to impose on it. People don't neatly fit into Autism or ADHD boxes, but rather, individuals have a unique cocktail of traits, each of which manifests in its own way. Some of those traits might lean more towards Autism – perhaps an overwhelming sensitivity to noise or a need for structure and predictability – while others seem to fall into ADHD territory, such as difficulties focusing on tasks or an impulsive need to chase novel experiences.

Yet time and again I come across people who exhibit a fascinating blend of both. These are the individuals who fall into the space we now call AuDHD, and with every new patient the question that keeps surfacing is whether AuDHD is a separate diagnosis or simply another point along a broader neurodevelopmental spectrum.

So, the question becomes: are these two conditions really separate at all, or are they simply different expressions of the same underlying neurodevelopmental differences?

The Argument for Seeing AuDHD as Part of a Neurodevelopmental Spectrum

The idea that Autism and ADHD could exist along a neurodevelopmental spectrum is a compelling one. For many of us in the field, this perspective shifts how we think about not only AuDHD but neurodevelopmental conditions more broadly. If we imagine Autism and ADHD not as two distinct conditions but as two ends of a shared spectrum, then we begin to understand how their traits can overlap, intermingle and present so uniquely in each individual.

In this view, AuDHD isn't a separate diagnosis but rather a point along the spectrum where traits of both Autism and ADHD come together. This makes sense when we consider how frequently these conditions co-occur. Studies have shown that more than 50 per cent of individuals diagnosed with Autism also meet the criteria for ADHD. That kind of overlap suggests that these are not entirely separate conditions. Instead, we may be looking at different expressions of the same neurodevelopmental differences, manifesting in different ways depending on the individual's unique brain wiring.

Take for example, a young woman I treated who was diagnosed with Autism in childhood. As she grew older, her struggles with focus, organisation and impulsivity became more apparent, leading to an ADHD diagnosis in her teens. But what struck me most was how interconnected her Autism and ADHD traits were. Her need for routine and predictability clashed with her impulsivity, making even the most mundane tasks a daily challenge. The same brain that craved predictability also sought constant novelty; a paradox that was difficult for her and her family to understand, let alone manage. Her story, like so many others, suggests that Autism and ADHD are not separate, but rather deeply intertwined, presenting unique challenges for those who live with both.

Genetic, Neurobiological and Behavioural Overlaps

The argument for AuDHD being part of a neurodevelopmental spectrum is not just theoretical; it is increasingly supported by genetic, neurobiological and behavioural research. In recent years genetic studies have revealed significant overlap between Autism and ADHD. Certain genetic variations, particularly those that affect how neurons in the brain communicate with each other, have been implicated in both conditions. This suggests that, at a genetic level, Autism and ADHD share common roots.

For example, research into synaptic functioning – how brain cells (neurons) connect and communicate – has shown that mutations in certain genes can lead to disruptions in these processes, which are thought to contribute to both Autism and ADHD. This is a crucial finding because it implies that the same underlying genetic mechanisms that lead to difficulties with social communication in Autism could also contribute to the attention and focus problems seen in ADHD.

But the overlap doesn't stop at genetics. Neuroimaging studies have shown that individuals with Autism and ADHD often display similar patterns of brain activity, particularly in areas related to attention, executive functioning and social cognition. This means that when we look at the brain through a neurobiological lens, the distinctions between Autism and ADHD are not as clear-cut as we once thought. Instead, we see that both conditions may arise from differences in how certain brain networks develop and function.

On a behavioural level, the overlap is even more apparent. Both Autism and ADHD can involve difficulties with attention, impulsivity and executive functioning. Many of my patients with Autism describe the challenges they face in focusing on tasks, managing their time and regulating their impulses – symptoms that would typically be associated with ADHD. Conversely, many of my patients with ADHD exhibit sensory sensitivities, social difficulties and a preference for routine – traits that we usually associate with Autism. This behavioural overlap is a key reason why AuDHD can be so difficult to diagnose, and why it often goes unrecognised for so long.

Shared Neurodevelopmental Pathways

If we zoom out and take a broader view, the case for shared neurodevelopmental pathways becomes even stronger. Neurodevelopmental conditions, by definition, arise from differences in how the brain develops. These differences can affect everything from synaptic pruning – the process by which unnecessary neural connections are eliminated during brain development – to how the brain processes sensory information and regulates behaviour.

What is becoming increasingly clear is that many of these processes are not specific to any one condition. Instead, they represent underlying differences in brain development that can lead to a range of neurodevelopmental traits. Some individuals may experience these traits in ways that fit the diagnostic criteria for Autism, while others may exhibit traits that are more consistent with ADHD. But for many, like those with AuDHD, the traits do not fit neatly into one category or the other. Instead, they represent a blending of both, where the lines between Autism and ADHD become blurred.

This is why many researchers are now advocating for a more dimensional view of neurodevelopmental conditions. Rather than seeing Autism and ADHD as separate boxes, this perspective allows us to think of these conditions as points along a shared spectrum of brain development. In this view, the brain differences that lead to Autism and ADHD are not so different after all; they are simply different expressions of the same underlying neurodevelopmental pathways.

Unique Challenges of Co-Occurrence

Acknowledging that Autism and ADHD may exist along a shared spectrum does not mean that the co-occurrence of these conditions is without its challenges. In fact, one of the most striking things I've observed in my work with individuals who have both Autism and ADHD is just how uniquely challenging it can be to live with both conditions.

The sensory sensitivities that often accompany Autism, for example, can make the hyperactivity and impulsivity of ADHD even more difficult to manage. One patient I worked with, a young man in his twenties, struggled with sensory overload in crowded spaces. Yet, his ADHD symptoms made him restless and impulsive, leading him to seek out those very same stimulating environments. The result was a constant push and pull between his need for sensory calm and his craving for novelty and excitement.

Another unique challenge arises from the social difficulties associated with both conditions. Individuals with Autism often struggle with understanding social cues and forming relationships, while those with ADHD may find it difficult to maintain focus during social interactions. When these two conditions are combined, it can lead to a situation where social interactions feel both overwhelming and fleeting, difficult to engage in and equally difficult to sustain. For many of my patients this has led to feelings of isolation and frustration, as they navigate a world that often seems to demand social skills they find difficult to master.

In children the challenges of living with both Autism and ADHD can manifest in school, where the need for focus, attention and social interaction can feel overwhelming. I've worked with many children who are easily distracted, struggle to follow instructions and have difficulty making friends, all of which can lead to academic and social difficulties. For these children, traditional educational settings may not provide the structure or support they need to thrive, and finding the right interventions can be a complex and ongoing process.

For adults the challenges of living with AuDHD often play out in the workplace or in relationships, where the demands of daily life can feel overwhelming. One of my adult patients, a highly intelligent and creative woman in her thirties, described how her ADHD made it difficult to focus on her work, while her Autism made it hard to navigate the social dynamics of her office. She often felt like she was falling behind, both in terms of her job performance and her social relationships, and this led to feelings of inadequacy and frustration. Like many individuals with AuDHD, she struggled to find the balance between her need for structure and her desire for stimulation – a balance that often seemed just out of reach.

AuDHD as a Separate Diagnosis: the Clinical Perspective

I remember a day, early in my career as a neurodevelopmental psychiatrist, when a mother brought her teenage son to my clinic. He had been diagnosed with Autism at a young age, but something about his presentation didn't quite fit the usual pattern. His mother described a constant restlessness in him, an inability to sit still or focus for more than a few minutes at a time. He would leap from task to task, starting projects and abandoning them halfway through. This wasn't just an issue of sensory overload or needing time alone to decompress – traits we often associate with Autism. This was something else: an impulsivity, a hyperactivity that didn't seem to belong to the realm of Autism alone.

As I listened, I realised what she was describing wasn't just Autism – it was ADHD, presenting alongside his Autism. Despite his original diagnosis, no one had ever considered ADHD as a possibility. They had viewed his difficulties with attention and focus as just part of the broader Autism picture. This young man had been grappling with two distinct neurodevelopmental conditions but only one had been acknowledged. In that moment, the need to recognise AuDHD as a unique diagnosis became glaringly clear.

Presenting AuDHD as a Unique Diagnosis

While many clinicians and researchers consider Autism and ADHD as two separate conditions that can co-occur, there is a growing argument for recognising AuDHD as a distinct clinical entity. This perspective doesn't deny the overlap between Autism and ADHD, but it suggests that when these conditions intersect, they create a unique profile that is more than the sum of its parts. Individuals with AuDHD experience challenges that are distinct from those who have Autism or ADHD alone. The interaction between these two conditions can amplify certain symptoms, mask others and create entirely new challenges that can't be fully understood by looking at Autism or ADHD in isolation.

For instance, a person with only Autism may have difficulties with social communication and sensory sensitivities, but they may still be able to focus intensely on tasks they enjoy. Conversely, someone with only ADHD might struggle with focus and impulsivity but navigate social situations with ease. But for individuals with AuDHD, the combination of these traits creates a unique experience. They may crave structure and routine, due to their Autism, but find it nearly impossible to maintain that structure because of their ADHD-related impulsivity. They may become overstimulated by sensory input but instead of retreating, as someone with Autism might, they may act impulsively, seeking out more stimulation – behaviours driven by their ADHD.

What we see in these individuals is not merely a combination of Autism and ADHD traits; it's a new profile entirely. The overlap of these conditions creates a distinct clinical picture that demands a tailored approach in diagnosis and treatment. Recognising AuDHD as a unique diagnosis would allow clinicians to better address the interactions between these conditions and develop more targeted interventions that consider both sets of symptoms in tandem.

Clinical Evidence: Why Distinct Recognition Matters

Over the years I've had the privilege of working with many individuals of all ages who present with both Autism and ADHD. What has struck me time and again is how standard treatments for either condition often fall short for those with AuDHD. Many patients with Autism benefit from behavioural therapies that focus on social skills, sensory integration and communication strategies. But for patients with AuDHD these therapies are often not enough. Their ADHD symptoms – impulsivity, inattention, hyperactivity – require different interventions, such as medication or cognitive behavioural therapy (CBT), targeting executive functioning skills. The problem is that many treatment plans are not designed to address both sets of symptoms, leaving patients feeling frustrated and misunderstood.

I recall working with an adult patient who had been diagnosed with Autism in childhood, followed by an ADHD diagnosis in her twenties. She had spent years in therapy, focusing on managing her sensory sensitivities and improving her social skills. Yet she continued to struggle with organising her time, completing tasks and controlling impulsive behaviours. It wasn't until we addressed her ADHD symptoms specifically, by incorporating medication and executive functioning strategies, that she began to see significant improvements in her day-to-day life.

This experience, and many others like it, has taught me that recognising AuDHD as a distinct diagnosis could lead to better outcomes for individuals. When we treat Autism and ADHD as two separate conditions, we risk missing the ways in which they interact. But when we recognise that these conditions can create a unique clinical picture, we open the door to more personalised treatments that address the full range of symptoms these individuals experience.

The DSM-5 and the Limits of Co-Diagnosis

Currently, the DSM-5 – the manual used by clinicians to diagnose mental health conditions – allows for the co-diagnosis of Autism and ADHD. This is a step forward from previous editions where clinicians were often hesitant to diagnose both conditions in the same individual. In this sense, the DSM-5 recognises that Autism and ADHD can coexist, but it still treats them as separate diagnoses, each with its own set of criteria and guidelines for treatment.

While the DSM-5's allowance for co-diagnosis is helpful, it falls short of acknowledging the distinct clinical challenges that arise when these conditions intersect. By treating Autism and ADHD as separate, the manual doesn't account for the unique difficulties faced by individuals with both conditions. It doesn't consider how the sensory overload of Autism might be exacerbated by the hyperactivity of ADHD, or how the rigidity of Autism might clash with the impulsivity of ADHD. As a result, clinicians are left trying to address each condition in isolation, often without a clear framework for understanding how the two interact.

This is where the case for AuDHD as a separate diagnosis becomes particularly important. If we acknowledge AuDHD as its own clinical entity, we can begin to develop diagnostic criteria that reflect the unique experiences of individuals with both autism and ADHD. This would not only improve the accuracy of diagnoses, but also lead to more comprehensive treatment plans that address the specific challenges of living with AuDHD.

My Role in Pioneering Dual Diagnosis Across the Lifespan

Over the course of my career, I have been fortunate to work with individuals across their lifespan, who present with both Autism and ADHD. Early on, I noticed that many of the adults I worked with had been misdiagnosed or had only received a partial diagnosis. Some had been diagnosed with Autism in childhood but struggled with undiagnosed ADHD symptoms well into adulthood. Others had been diagnosed with ADHD as children but had not received an Autism diagnosis until much later in life. In both cases, these individuals were left feeling like something had been missed, as though their struggles were not fully understood or addressed.

This realisation led me to focus on dual diagnosis – the recognition that many individuals live with both Autism and ADHD, and that these conditions often interact in complex ways. I began to advocate for a more integrated approach to diagnosis and treatment, one that considers the full range of symptoms these individuals experience rather than treating each condition in isolation. Over time, I have worked with countless patients to help them understand how their Autism and ADHD interact, and I have seen first-hand the transformative impact that a dual diagnosis can have.

One of the most rewarding aspects of my work has been helping patients who have struggled for years without a full understanding of their condition. For many, receiving a dual diagnosis has been a relief: a way to make sense of their lifelong challenges and finally receive the support they need. It has been a privilege to walk alongside them as they begin to understand their neurodevelopmental profile more fully and see the positive changes that come from receiving targeted, personalised treatments.

As I continue my work in this area, I am hopeful that the recognition of AuDHD as a distinct clinical entity will continue to grow. The intersection of Autism and ADHD is a complex and often misunderstood space, but with continued research, clinical practice and advocacy, we can move towards a more nuanced understanding of how these conditions interact and how best to support those who live with both.

Chapter 7: Towards a Better Understanding of AuDHD

Whether we view AuDHD as a distinct entity or as part of a broader neurodevelopmental spectrum, what matters most is that we recognise the unique challenges faced by individuals with both Autism and ADHD. By doing so, we can develop more effective diagnostic tools and treatment plans that address the full scope of their needs.

In my own practice, I have seen the profound impact that recognition and treatment can have on individuals with AuDHD. When we acknowledge the complexity of their neurodevelopmental profile, we offer them the opportunity not only to better understand themselves but also to access the support and interventions they need to thrive. My hope is that, as we move forward in our understanding of AuDHD, we will continue to push the boundaries of our diagnostic frameworks and clinical practices, ensuring that no one is left behind in their journey towards understanding and healing.

Challenges of Co-Occurrence

There's a unique tension that comes with the co-occurrence of Autism and ADHD, one that plays out not only in the consulting room but also in the everyday lives of individuals, families and clinicians alike. This tension exists because managing both conditions together is rarely as straightforward as addressing them separately. It's in this space, where Autism and ADHD meet, that the complexity of treatment, understanding and care becomes most apparent.

I remember a particular family that came to see me: the parents exhausted; their teenage son restless and disengaged. He had been diagnosed with Autism at a young age and had spent years in therapies focused on managing his sensory sensitivities and social communication difficulties. But as he entered adolescence, his behaviour became more erratic – he was impulsive, inattentive and easily distracted. His school reported that he couldn't focus in class, often wandering around or interrupting his peers. Despite this, his previous clinicians had chalked it all up to his Autism, attributing these traits to the natural progression of his condition. As I listened to his story, it became clear that something else was at play: this wasn't just Autism. It was ADHD, interwoven with his Autism in a way that made it difficult to separate one condition from the other.

This family, like so many others, was facing the challenges of co-diagnosis – the intersection of two distinct but overlapping neurodevelopmental conditions that create a complex, and often confusing, clinical picture.

Managing Both ASD and ADHD: the Challenges for Patients and Clinicians

When Autism and ADHD co-occur, they create a unique set of challenges that go beyond what we typically see in individuals with just one condition. For patients, these challenges manifest in ways that can feel contradictory. A person with Autism might need structure and routine to feel safe and grounded, while their ADHD makes it difficult for them to maintain that structure. They may struggle with sensory overload, but their ADHD-driven impulsivity might push them towards environments that are overstimulating. For many of my patients this push and pull between the two conditions creates a sense of internal chaos, where their needs seem to conflict with each other, leaving them feeling frustrated and misunderstood.

For clinicians the challenge is often one of navigation. Autism and ADHD, when they occur together, do not simply exist side by side – they interact, often amplifying or masking each other's symptoms. This makes it difficult to determine which behaviours are driven by Autism and which by ADHD. A child who fidgets and struggles to sit still might be doing so because of their ADHD, but they could also be experiencing sensory discomfort from their Autism. Similarly, difficulties with attention and focus might stem from ADHD, but they could also be related to the repetitive thoughts and rigid thinking patterns common in Autism.

This interplay between conditions requires a nuanced understanding of both Autism and ADHD, as well as the ability to adapt treatment plans to address the specific challenges that arise when the two coexist. Unfortunately, not many clinicians are trained to treat these conditions together, leading to a fragmented approach that fails to address the full scope of an individual's needs.

Complex Treatments: Why These Complexities Matter

The co-occurrence of Autism and ADHD often leads to more complex treatment plans, and while complexity can be challenging, it is also necessary. The reality is that individuals with both conditions require multiple layers of intervention; there is no one-size-fits-all solution. This complexity arises because Autism and ADHD need different approaches to treatment, and when these conditions occur together, the treatment plan must address both.

For example, an individual with Autism might benefit from behavioural therapies focused on social skills, sensory processing and communication. But if they also have ADHD, these therapies will only address part of the problem. Their inattention, impulsivity and hyperactivity need to be managed as well, often through medication and cognitive behavioural strategies aimed at improving executive functioning. The challenge is finding the right balance, ensuring that the treatment for one condition doesn't exacerbate the other.

I've seen this balance play out in a number of my patients, particularly in adults who have spent years being treated for one condition while the other remained undiagnosed. One patient, a woman in her forties, had been diagnosed with Autism in her twenties but had never received an ADHD diagnosis, despite struggling with chronic disorganisation, impulsivity and difficulties maintaining focus. Her Autism therapies had helped her manage her social and sensory challenges, but they did nothing for her ADHD symptoms. It wasn't until we introduced stimulant medication and executive functioning coaching that she began to see real improvements in her ability to manage day-to-day life. But even then, the challenge was ensuring that the stimulant medication didn't exacerbate her sensory sensitivities – a common issue in individuals with both Autism and ADHD.

This is why the complexity of treatment matters: without addressing both conditions, patients are left with incomplete care. They may see some improvements, but the full picture of their neurodevelopmental needs remains unmet. By recognising the complexity of AuDHD and creating integrated treatment plans, we can ensure that individuals receive the care they need to thrive.

Misdiagnoses: When One Condition Overshadows the Other

One of the most significant challenges of co-diagnosis is the risk of misdiagnosis. When Autism and ADHD co-occur, it is common for one condition to overshadow the other, leading to incomplete or incorrect diagnoses. This can happen for a number of reasons, but one of the most common is that Autism and ADHD share overlapping traits, such as difficulties with attention, impulsivity and social interactions. This overlap can make it difficult for clinicians to tease apart the specific symptoms of each condition.

People with AuDHD are also misdiagnosed with conditions like Social Anxiety, Complex Trauma, Personality Disorders, Bipolar Affective Disorder or Cyclothymia.

In some cases, individuals are diagnosed with Autism at a young age, and their ADHD symptoms are attributed to the same condition. This was the case with the teenage boy I mentioned earlier – his impulsivity and inattention were seen as stereotypical of his Autism, and no one considered ADHD as a possibility. It wasn't until his behaviours became more disruptive that the ADHD diagnosis was considered, years after he had already been struggling with the condition.

Conversely, I have worked with adults who were diagnosed with ADHD in childhood but never received an Autism diagnosis, despite exhibiting clear traits of the condition. One patient, a man in his thirties, had been diagnosed with ADHD as a child and had spent his life managing his symptoms with medication. But he continued to struggle with social communication, rigid thinking and sensory sensitivities – all hallmarks of Autism. It wasn't until he sought a second opinion in adulthood that he was diagnosed with Autism, finally providing him with the clarity he needed to understand his full neurodevelopmental profile.

It is quite common for individuals with ADHD, even those well-managed on medication, to express concerns about intermittent low mood and anxiety. In many cases, this is the unveiling of underlying autistic traits. I take the time to carefully explain the complex interaction between Autism and ADHD, including where the symptoms overlap, to help patients better understand the full picture of their neurodiversity.

These misdiagnoses occur because clinicians often focus on the more prominent condition, overlooking the subtler symptoms of the other. In the case of Autism, the social and sensory challenges can overshadow the impulsivity and inattention of ADHD, while in the case of ADHD, the hyperactivity and disorganisation can mask the social difficulties and sensory sensitivities of Autism. This is why it is so important for clinicians to be aware of the possibility of co-diagnosis and to consider both conditions when assessing patients.

The Impact on Families, Schooling and Social Services

The challenges of co-diagnosis extend beyond the individual to their families, schools and social services. For families, navigating the dual diagnosis of Autism and ADHD can be overwhelming. Parents may struggle to understand how to meet the diverse needs of their child, particularly when the strategies that work for one condition don't seem to work for the other. A child with Autism might need calm, structured environments, but their ADHD symptoms may make it difficult for them to maintain focus or follow through with routines. This can leave parents feeling frustrated and unsure of how to support their child effectively.

In schools, the dual diagnosis of Autism and ADHD presents its own set of challenges. Teachers may struggle to provide the individualised support that these students need, particularly when the strategies for managing Autism (such as providing routine and structure) clash with the strategies for managing ADHD (such as allowing for movement and flexibility). This can lead to academic difficulties, social isolation and behavioural challenges, all of which can impact the student's ability to thrive in the classroom.

Social services also play a role in supporting individuals with AuDHD, but they often face similar challenges. Many social service programmes are designed to address either Autism or ADHD, but not both. This can leave families and individuals without access to the full range of support they need, particularly when it comes to therapies, educational resources and social-skills training. The dual diagnosis of Autism and ADHD requires a more holistic approach to care – one that takes into account the complex needs of individuals with both conditions and provides integrated services that address those needs.

Embracing Complexity for Better Outcomes

The co-diagnosis of Autism and ADHD presents a unique set of challenges, for the individuals living with these conditions and for the clinicians, families and social services that support them. But these challenges also represent an opportunity. By recognising the complexity of AuDHD and embracing the need for integrated, personalised care, we can begin to provide more effective treatments and support for those who live with both Autism and ADHD.

For many of my patients, receiving a dual diagnosis has been the key to unlocking their full potential. It has allowed them to understand the complexities of their neurodevelopmental profile and to access the treatments and strategies that address the full range of their needs. As we continue to advance our understanding of AuDHD, it is my hope that more individuals will have the opportunity to receive the holistic, integrated care they need to thrive, both in their personal lives and in the wider world.

Research Evidence: Genetics, Neurobiology and Behavioural Studies

In the journey of understanding how the brain works, especially in the context of Autism Spectrum Condition (ASC) and Attention Deficit Hyperactivity Disorder

(ADHD), I've often found myself reflecting on the richness of human diversity. Each brain is a universe of its own, and for those with AuDHD – the intersection of Autism and ADHD – this universe is especially complex. As a neurodevelopmental psychiatrist, I've spent years sifting through research, listening to the lived experiences of patients, and observing first-hand the ways in which Autism and ADHD manifest. The deeper we delve into the genetics, neurobiology and behavioural studies surrounding these conditions, the clearer it becomes that their overlap is not accidental or coincidental. Instead, it hints at shared pathways in the brain, which raises both new questions and exciting possibilities.

A Genetic Foundation: Shared Roots of ASD and ADHD

The first step in understanding the co-occurrence of Autism and ADHD is to explore the genetic evidence. One of the most striking revelations from recent research is that these conditions share a significant number of genetic risk factors. As we sequence genomes and uncover the blueprints of human development, we see clear connections between the genes involved in brain development and the regulation of neurotransmitters in both Autism and ADHD.

It wasn't long ago that these two conditions were thought to be entirely separate, but today, genetic studies paint a different picture. For instance, variations in genes like DRD4, which is linked to dopamine receptors, and DAT1, responsible for dopamine transport, are found in both individuals with ADHD and those with Autism. These genes play a critical role in the brain's reward system and executive functioning – two areas that are often impaired in both Autism and ADHD.

A study published in *Nature Genetics* highlighted this overlap by showing how certain genetic mutations affect synaptic transmission – the way neurons communicate. In both conditions, these mutations can lead to disruptions in brain signalling, particularly in areas that control attention, impulsivity and social interactions. This shared genetic framework suggests that Autism and ADHD may stem from similar neurodevelopmental disruptions, with slight variations determining the exact nature of the symptoms.

In twin studies, scientists have found that when one twin is diagnosed with Autism, there is a significantly increased likelihood that the other twin will have ADHD, and vice versa. This familial clustering of the two conditions supports the idea that they are genetically linked rather than entirely separate phenomena. It also sheds light on why many families, when receiving a diagnosis for one child, may later discover that other siblings also present traits of Autism, ADHD, or both. These findings have changed how we think about the brain's development, emphasising the genetic interplay that creates the diverse range of experiences we see in individuals with Autism and ADHD.

Neurobiology: Mapping the Brain's Overlap

While genetics provide the foundation, it is through neuroscientific studies that we can begin to visualise the actual workings of the brain in individuals with both Autism and ADHD. Neuroimaging has been a powerful tool in this regard, allowing us to see in real-time how different brain regions are activated and how they communicate, or fail to communicate.

One of the most fascinating discoveries in recent years has been the role of the prefrontal cortex: the part of the brain responsible for executive functions like decision-making, impulse control and focusing attention. In individuals with ADHD, the prefrontal cortex often shows delayed development or reduced activity, which explains why they struggle with tasks that require sustained attention or inhibition of impulses. But here's where it gets interesting: similar disruptions in the prefrontal cortex have been found in individuals with Autism, particularly in those who struggle with rigidity of thought and executive dysfunction.

Neuroimaging studies have mapped out other shared brain regions, such as the anterior cingulate cortex (ACC), which is crucial for emotion regulation and error monitoring. In ADHD, the ACC is often underactive, leading to difficulties in recognising and correcting mistakes. In Autism, the ACC is linked to the challenges individuals face in processing emotional and social information. The fact that this same brain region is implicated in both conditions suggests that Autism and ADHD may represent different expressions of the same neurobiological vulnerabilities.

Another key player in both conditions is the dopaminergic system, and particularly the pathways involving dopamine – a neurotransmitter critical for motivation, reward and attention. In ADHD, dopamine dysregulation leads to the well-documented difficulties with focus and impulsivity. In Autism, abnormalities in dopamine signalling may explain the intense focus on specific interests and the repetitive behaviours that are characteristic of the condition. By studying the dopaminergic system in individuals with both Autism and ADHD, neuroscientists are beginning to piece together how disruptions in this system can lead to the dual presentation of traits seen in AuDHD.

These neurobiological overlaps underscore the idea that Autism and ADHD are not just coincidental co-occurrences but are deeply intertwined conditions. They share the same neural circuitry, which is why individuals with AuDHD often experience a unique blend of challenges related to both social communication and executive functioning.

Behavioural and Cognitive Studies: Everyday Interactions of ASD and ADHD

While genetics and neurobiology give us the theoretical framework, it is through behavioural and cognitive studies that we see how these conditions play out in everyday life. One of the hallmarks of AuDHD is the internal conflict between the needs and tendencies of Autism and those of ADHD.

For instance, a child with Autism may crave structure and predictability, finding comfort in routine. However, their ADHD traits may drive a desire for novelty and stimulation, leading to a constant tension between the need for stability and the impulsive urge to seek out new experiences. This creates a dynamic where the individual is pulled in opposing directions, making it difficult to find equilibrium. In behavioural studies, we often see this tension manifest in disruptions to executive functioning, such as difficulty organising tasks, following through on plans and managing time effectively.

The Need for More Research: AuDHD's Place in Clinical Practice

Despite the advances in our understanding of how Autism and ADHD overlap, there is still much we do not know about AuDHD. One of the key challenges facing clinicians today is how to classify and treat AuDHD effectively. Current diagnostic systems, such as the DSM-5, allow for the co-diagnosis of Autism and ADHD, but they do not provide clear guidance on how to address the unique needs of individuals with both conditions.

More research is needed to determine whether AuDHD should be recognised as a distinct clinical entity, separate from Autism and ADHD, or whether it should be considered part of a broader neurodevelopmental spectrum. This research must explore not only the genetic and neurobiological overlaps but also how these conditions interact in different contexts, such as school, work and social environments. We also need more studies that investigate the long-term outcomes for individuals with AuDHD, particularly in terms of how they navigate adulthood, where the demands of independence and social interaction become more pronounced.

The research evidence we have thus far suggests that individuals with AuDHD require tailored interventions that address the unique combination of traits they experience. This may involve a mix of behavioural therapies, medication and supportive services that are designed to meet the specific needs of individuals with both Autism and ADHD. However, to develop these interventions, we must first gain a deeper understanding of how these conditions interact at every level, from the genetic to the social.

Practical Implications of Recognising AuDHD

I have often found myself sitting with patients, listening to them describe a life of struggle and confusion, one that has been shaped by a diagnosis of Autism Spectrum Condition (ASC) or Attention Deficit Hyperactivity Disorder (ADHD) – or sometimes, neither. Yet, the words they use to describe their experiences reflect the challenges of living with both conditions. They tell me stories of feeling like their brain is constantly pulling them in different directions, where their need for structure (a hallmark of Autism) is undermined by their impulsivity (a key feature of ADHD). Or they speak of their deep, intense focus on particular interests, while simultaneously struggling to sustain attention on tasks that don't hold their attention.

These stories echo through my practice, and they highlight the need to recognise AuDHD not just as a theoretical construct, but as a reality that affects the lives of many individuals. The practical implications of recognising AuDHD, whether we consider it part of a neurodevelopmental spectrum or a separate diagnosis, are profound. It matters because how we diagnose and define AuDHD will shape how we treat, support and accommodate those who live with it.

Why It Matters to Recognise AuDHD

At its core, recognising AuDHD is about validation – for both patients and clinicians. For individuals who have lived their entire lives feeling as though they don't fit neatly into the categories of Autism or ADHD, recognising AuDHD provides a sense of clarity. It allows them to understand that their experiences are real, valid and worthy of attention. It acknowledges that their struggles are not isolated or unrelated, but rather, the result of a unique combination of traits from both conditions.

From a clinical perspective, recognising AuDHD is equally important. As we've seen throughout the research and clinical practice, Autism and ADHD frequently co-occur, with more than 50 per cent of individuals diagnosed with Autism also meeting the criteria for ADHD. This overlap is not just a curiosity; it's a reality that affects diagnosis, treatment and outcomes. By recognising AuDHD, we move away from the rigid boundaries that separate Autism and ADHD, and towards a more holistic view of neurodevelopmental conditions. This shift allows clinicians to better address the full range of symptoms that individuals with AuDHD experience, rather than focusing on one condition at the expense of the other.

But beyond diagnosis, recognising AuDHD is about equity. It does not matter whether it's part of the spectrum or a separate diagnosis. It ensures that individuals with dual diagnoses receive the same level of attention, care and support as those with singular diagnoses. Without recognition, the risk is that people with AuDHD will continue to slip through the cracks, their needs overlooked because they don't fit the traditional mould of Autism or ADHD. Recognition means opening new pathways for understanding, treatment and support.

The Impact on Treatment Options: Medications, Therapies and Support Services

One of the most significant practical implications of recognising AuDHD lies in how it changes our approach to treatment. Traditional treatments for Autism and

ADHD have evolved separately, each with its own set of strategies, medications and therapies. Autism treatments often focus on social-skills training, sensory integration therapies and behavioural interventions designed to improve communication and reduce repetitive behaviours. ADHD treatments, on the other hand, rely heavily on stimulant medications to address inattention and impulsivity, alongside cognitive behavioural therapy (CBT) aimed at improving executive functioning.

For individuals with AuDHD, these separate treatment pathways are often insufficient. Their ADHD symptoms may respond well to stimulant medications, but those same medications can sometimes exacerbate their Autism-related sensory sensitivities or increase anxiety. Conversely, while social-skills training may help with their Autism, it may not address the impulsivity or disorganisation caused by ADHD. Recognising AuDHD allows us to integrate treatment plans, combining the most effective elements of both Autism and ADHD therapies in ways that cater to the specific needs of the individual.

In practice, this means more personalised medication regimens. For example, non-stimulant medications like Guanfacine or Atomoxetine, or slow-release stimulants which have been shown to reduce ADHD symptoms, may be better suited for individuals with sensory sensitivities. In some cases, combining low-dose stimulants with behavioural therapies may strike the right balance, helping individuals to manage their ADHD symptoms without worsening their Autism-related challenges.

Beyond medications, recognising AuDHD also opens the door to more comprehensive support services. Individuals with AuDHD often need a combination of therapies that address both social communication difficulties and executive dysfunction. This might mean working with occupational therapists who specialise in sensory processing, alongside executive functioning coaches who can help with time management, organisation and task initiation. It's this multi-pronged approach that will lead to the best outcomes, ensuring that all aspects of the individual's neurodevelopmental profile are addressed.

Changing Our Approach to Schooling, Workplace Accommodations and Societal Views on Neurodiversity

When we recognise AuDHD, the implications extend far beyond clinical settings. It changes how we approach schooling, workplace accommodations and even how society views neurodiversity.

In schools, children with both Autism and ADHD often face challenges that are not adequately addressed by traditional special education programmes. A child with Autism may benefit from structured routines and clear expectations, but their ADHD symptoms may make it difficult for them to sit still or stay focused for long periods. Without recognition of their dual diagnosis, these children can end up feeling frustrated, misunderstood or even punished for behaviours that are beyond their control.

I once worked with a family whose son, diagnosed with both Autism and ADHD, struggled in a mainstream classroom. His teachers were well-versed in Autism supports, providing him with visual schedules and allowing for sensory breaks. But his ADHD symptoms were largely ignored, leading to constant disruptions in class. He was labelled as having a 'behaviour problem' because he couldn't sit still or pay attention, despite his teachers' efforts to accommodate his Autism. It wasn't until we developed a plan that addressed both conditions, incorporating frequent movement breaks, clear expectations and strategies for managing impulsivity, that he began to thrive academically.

In the workplace, individuals with AuDHD face similar challenges. Many workplaces are beginning to embrace neurodiversity, but accommodations often focus on singular diagnoses. For example, a person with Autism may benefit from noise-cancelling headphones or flexible work hours to manage sensory sensitivities, but their ADHD symptoms may require structured deadlines or regular feedback to stay on track. Without recognition of their dual diagnosis, individuals with AuDHD may find it difficult to advocate for the full range of accommodations they need.

By recognising AuDHD, we can create workplaces that are more inclusive and flexible, allowing individuals to succeed without having to choose between managing their Autism or ADHD symptoms. This shift in how we approach neurodiversity can lead to more innovative workplace policies, such as individualised accommodation plans that take into account the unique needs of those with dual diagnoses.

On a broader societal level, recognising AuDHD contributes to a more nuanced understanding of neurodiversity. It challenges the notion that people with Autism or ADHD fit into neat categories, and it encourages us to view the brain as a spectrum of experiences. This perspective fosters greater acceptance and compassion for the diverse ways in which people navigate the world, ultimately reducing the stigma associated with neurodevelopmental conditions.

Personal Anecdotes: the Power of a Dual Diagnosis

I'll never forget a patient I worked with years ago: a woman in her early twenties who had been diagnosed with ADHD as a child. She had spent years trying to manage her symptoms – taking medication for her inattention and impulsivity, as well as attending therapy to improve her executive functioning – but something always felt off. She struggled in social situations, often feeling out of step with her peers. Loud noises and busy environments overwhelmed her, and she found comfort in routines and repetitive tasks – traits that didn't quite fit the ADHD profile.

When we explored the possibility of Autism, it was as if a lightbulb went off for her. She had always felt like there was more to her story than just ADHD, and receiving the dual diagnosis of Autism and ADHD gave her the clarity she had been searching for. With this new understanding, we were able to develop a treatment plan that addressed both conditions, incorporating sensory supports, social communication strategies, and adjustments to her ADHD medication. For the first time she felt seen and understood.

Another patient, a middle-aged man who had struggled with both social interactions and impulsivity his entire life, had been diagnosed with Autism in his early twenties. He had developed coping strategies to manage his sensory sensitivities and difficulty with change, but he continued to have trouble focusing on tasks, managing his time and controlling his impulses. When he was finally diagnosed with ADHD in his forties, everything clicked. His impulsivity and inattention weren't just part of his Autism; they were symptoms of ADHD, and with the right treatment, he was able to make significant improvements in his daily functioning.

These personal anecdotes are just two examples of the countless individuals who have benefited from a dual diagnosis. For them, recognising AuDHD was the key to unlocking their potential and finding the support they needed to thrive. It's a reminder that when we take the time to understand the full complexity of someone's neurodevelopmental profile, we can provide them with the tools to lead more fulfilling, empowered lives.

A Call for Recognition

As a neurodevelopmental psychiatrist, I've seen firsthand the transformative power of recognising AuDHD. Whether we view it as part of a neurodevelopmental spectrum or as a separate diagnosis, what matters most is that we acknowledge the unique challenges faced by individuals with both Autism and ADHD. By doing so, we open the door to more effective treatments, more inclusive schools and workplaces, and a society that truly values neurodiversity.

The practical implications of recognising AuDHD are profound. It changes how we approach treatment, allowing for more personalised and integrated care. It reshapes how we think about schooling and workplace accommodations, ensuring that individuals with dual diagnoses receive the support they need to succeed. And most importantly, it gives individuals with AuDHD the validation they deserve, helping them understand that their experiences are real, complex and worthy of attention.

Future Directions: Where Do We Go from Here?

As I sit here, reflecting on the many years I've spent working with individuals who live at the intersection of Autism and ADHD, I find myself both inspired by how far we've come and eager for what lies ahead. The journey of understanding AuDHD has been one of gradual discovery, with each new piece of research, each patient I've met, adding a layer of complexity to this already intricate picture. And yet, there is still so much we don't know. The future of AuDHD research and clinical practice holds immense potential, and if we are to truly support those who live with these dual diagnoses, we must embrace the challenges and opportunities that lie ahead.

The Future of AuDHD Research: Unlocking the Brain's Secrets

One of the most exciting frontiers in understanding AuDHD lies in the continued exploration of the brain's mysteries. We have already made significant strides in understanding the genetic, neurobiological and behavioural links between Autism and ADHD, but there is still much to be uncovered. As technology advances, so too does our ability to map the brain with greater precision and detail. In the coming years I believe we will see breakthroughs in neuroimaging and genetic research that will shed light on exactly how the brains of individuals with AuDHD are wired and how we can better tailor treatments to their specific needs.

For instance, as we refine our understanding of the dopaminergic system – the network of neurotransmitters that regulates motivation, attention and reward – we may discover more about how dopamine dysregulation contributes to the symptoms of both Autism and ADHD. This could lead to new medications that target these pathways more precisely, offering relief for individuals whose current treatment options may be limited or ineffective. Similarly, advances in functional MRI and other neuroimaging techniques may allow us to better understand the interactions between the prefrontal cortex, anterior cingulate cortex, and other brain regions involved in executive functioning, social cognition and emotional regulation.

Beyond neurobiology, the future of AuDHD research must also include a more comprehensive approach to understanding how these conditions interact with one another in everyday life. We need long-term studies that follow individuals with dual diagnoses from childhood through adulthood, tracking their developmental trajectories, educational and professional outcomes, and mental health. These studies will not only provide valuable data on how Autism and ADHD evolve over time, but also guide the development of more holistic treatment plans that address the unique needs of individuals at different life stages.

A Call for More Nuanced Diagnostic Frameworks in Psychiatry

As we move forward, one of the most pressing needs in the field of psychiatry is the development of more nuanced diagnostic frameworks that capture the complexity of

AuDHD. Currently, our diagnostic systems, such as the DSM-5, allow for the co-diagnosis of Autism and ADHD, but they do not provide clear guidance on how to distinguish between the overlapping symptoms of these conditions or how to best treat individuals who present with both.

It's time for us to move beyond the binary thinking that has traditionally shaped psychiatric diagnoses. Rather than viewing Autism and ADHD as distinct and separate entities, we need a framework that reflects the spectrum of neurodevelopmental experiences. This would mean recognising that individuals with AuDHD may present with a unique combination of traits from both conditions and that their symptoms may interact in ways that create entirely new challenges.

A more dimensional approach to diagnosis would allow clinicians to capture the full range of an individual's neurodevelopmental profile, rather than trying to fit them into pre-existing categories. This would not only improve the accuracy of diagnoses but also ensure that individuals receive the right interventions at the right time. For example, a child with both Autism and ADHD may benefit from early interventions that address their social communication challenges, alongside strategies for managing inattention and impulsivity. As that child grows into adolescence and adulthood, their treatment plan would evolve to address the changing demands of school, work and social relationships.

Nuanced diagnostic frameworks also have the potential to reduce misdiagnosis and underdiagnosis, which are all too common in individuals with AuDHD. By providing clinicians with clearer guidelines on how to recognise and treat dual diagnoses, we can prevent individuals from being left without the support they need, simply because they don't fit neatly into the existing diagnostic categories.

Advocating for Better Recognition and Support for AuDHD

While the future of AuDHD research and diagnostic frameworks is promising, we cannot afford to wait for these advancements to materialise before taking action. The reality is that many individuals with AuDHD are already struggling in a system that doesn't fully understand or support them. As clinicians, patients and advocates, we must work together to ensure that better recognition and support for AuDHD becomes a priority.

For clinicians, this means actively seeking out continuing education on dual diagnoses, as well as advocating for more integrated care models that address both Autism and ADHD simultaneously. It means recognising that individuals with AuDHD often require multidisciplinary support, including input from neurologists, psychiatrists, psychologists, occupational therapists and social workers. By fostering a more collaborative approach to care, we can ensure that patients with AuDHD receive the comprehensive treatment they need to thrive.

Patients and families can also play a crucial role in advocating for better recognition and support. By sharing their experiences and raising awareness about the challenges of living with both Autism and ADHD, they can help to reduce the stigma that often surrounds dual diagnoses. In my practice, I have seen the power of advocacy first-hand. One patient, a young woman diagnosed with AuDHD in her twenties, became a vocal advocate for dual diagnosis awareness after struggling for years without a proper diagnosis. Through her efforts, she has helped countless others in her community to understand that it's possible to live a fulfilling life with both Autism and ADHD, as long as the right supports are in place.

At a societal level, we need to push for policies that promote inclusive education, workplace accommodations, and access to mental health care for individuals with dual diagnoses. This includes advocating for schools to provide individualised education plans (IEPs) that address both the social communication challenges of Autism and the executive functioning difficulties of ADHD. It also means ensuring that workplaces adopt policies that accommodate neurodiverse employees, allowing them to thrive without compromising their mental health.

Concluding Thoughts: How Far We've Come and Where We Need to Go Next

As I look back on my years of working with individuals who live with AuDHD, I am struck by how far we have come in understanding the complexities of this dual diagnosis. When I first began my career, Autism and ADHD were largely viewed as separate conditions, and the idea of a shared neurodevelopmental spectrum was still in its infancy. Today, we have a much deeper understanding of how these conditions overlap, interact and shape the lives of those who experience them.

But as much progress as we've made, there is still a long way to go. The future of AuDHD research holds the potential to unlock new insights into the brain's development, leading to more effective treatments and better outcomes for individuals with dual diagnoses. At the same time, we must continue to push for more nuanced diagnostic frameworks that capture the full range of neurodevelopmental diversity, ensuring that no one is left behind because their symptoms don't fit neatly into existing categories.

As clinicians, patients and advocates, we have a responsibility to work towards a future where individuals with AuDHD are fully understood and supported. This means embracing the complexity of dual diagnoses, advocating for more inclusive policies and continuing to push the boundaries of what we know about the brain. By doing so, we can ensure that individuals with AuDHD not only survive but thrive, leading fulfilling, empowered lives where their unique strengths are celebrated, and their challenges are met with compassion and care.

The work we do today to recognise and support individuals with AuDHD will lay the foundation for a future where neurodiversity is not just accepted but embraced. And that is a future worth striving for.

As I conclude this book, I feel a sense of gratitude. For all the struggles, the confusion and the self-doubt, AuDHD has also given me strengths I wouldn't trade for anything. It has made me resilient, creative and determined to make a difference in the world. And through my work, I hope to continue spreading the message that every brain, every neurodivergent mind, deserves to be understood, celebrated and supported.

Acknowledgements

This book is dedicated to the journey of discovery, shaped by the people who have made it possible. I owe my deepest gratitude to my father, a brilliant mechanical engineer and a fellow AuDHDer, who has been my guiding light in more ways than I can express. He was the most intelligent person I have ever known, a masterful storyteller who wove context into every conversation. His unconventional thinking inspired me to see the world differently, fight for what is right and never settle for easy answers. Thank you, Abu, for teaching me to think beyond the obvious.

To my mother, whose progressive mindset and resilience made my upbringing in a small town a powerful foundation for my journey.

To my lovely wife Nadia, thank you for giving me the space to pursue the causes that resonate within me and for creating a tranquil, supportive environment that allows me to thrive. You have been my calm amid storms.

My sons, Farhaan and Sameer, and my nephew Zaigham, thank you for picking up the pieces when I needed it most – your love and laughter revitalise me at the end of each day. To my sister Zara, who has tirelessly managed things back home, making it possible for me to focus on my work here with peace of mind – thank you for your unwavering support and for holding it all together.

To my paternal grandfather, who instilled in me a love for storytelling and showed me that compassion is at the heart of connection – your legacy lives on in every word I write. You taught me that stories are bridges, connecting generations and ideas, and for that, I am eternally grateful.

I am also indebted to my first teacher, Miss Nighat Shamim, whose enthusiasm for biological sciences sparked a lifelong fascination in me. My mentor, Dr Prem Mahadun, showed me the essence of true leadership and how to cultivate a workplace that fosters growth and learning. His guidance has been invaluable in my journey.

To my dear friends, Fleur and Suzy, your support in my neurodiversity work and your unwavering encouragement have meant the world to me. To my cherished mentees and friends, Hina Rehman and Sandhya, and to my friends Fayyaz and Anwar – thank you for being there every step of the way, urging me to reach further and think deeper.

I am grateful to my colleagues and friends at Oxleas NHS Foundation Trust, for their faith in my vision and for supporting my work in a way that allowed me the freedom to grow, explore and realise my aspirations. Thank you for fostering an environment where autonomy and trust are the cornerstones.

A heartfelt thanks to my extended family – Bari Phoopho, Uncle Saqib, Amma, Baba, Salman, Sobana, Shaheer and Umair – and my esteemed colleagues Dr Bhuwan Roy, Dr Ajay Bhatnagar, Dr Tharangini Murugaiyan, Dr Saadia Muzaffar, Dr Mohammed Gul, and Steve Grange. Your continued support and encouragement have been a constant source of strength and inspiration.

I am most grateful to my patients, who have entrusted me with their stories, their struggles and their triumphs. Their courage in opening up has been my greatest source of learning and growth. My patients are my living textbooks, offering insights that no literature could replicate. Their journeys and experiences have profoundly enriched my understanding, and this book would not have been possible without the invaluable lessons they have taught me.

Lastly, to Martina O'Sullivan, my editor, thank you for seeing potential in this project and for your patience, encouragement and unwavering belief in my vision. You reached out when I needed that final push, guiding me to bring forth my best, and you stood by every draft and revision with boundless patience.

This work is a tapestry woven from your love, support and belief in me. Thank you, each of you, for being part of this journey.

Further Reading

Storytelling/Lived Experience:

Willey, LH. *Pretending to be Normal: Living with Asperger's Syndrome (Expanded Edition)*. Jessica Kingsley Publishers; 2014 Sep 21.

Grandin T, Panek R. *The Autistic Brain: Thinking Across the Spectrum*. Houghton Mifflin Harcourt; 2013.

Higashida, N. *The Reason I Jump: The Inner Voice of a Thirteen-Year-Old Boy with Autism*. Knopf Canada; 2013 Aug 27.

Maté, G. *Scattered Minds: The Origins and Healing of Attention Deficit Disorder*. Vintage Canada; 2011 Jul 27.

Middleton, E. *Unmasked: The Ultimate Guide to ADHD, Autism and Neurodivergence*. Penguin Life; 26 Oct 23.

Price, D. Unmasking autism: The power of embracing our hidden neurodiversity. Hachette UK; 2022 Apr 7.

Gooding, L. *Wonderfully Wired Brains: An Introduction to the World of Neurodiversity*. DK Children; 4 May 23.

Surman, C, Bilkey, T, Weintraub K. *FAST MINDS: How to Thrive if You Have ADHD (or Think You Might)*. Penguin; 2014 Jun 3.

Brown, TE. *Smart but Stuck: Emotions in Teens and Adults with ADHD*. John Wiley & Sons; 2014 Feb 3.

Professionals:

Banaschewski, T, Coghill, D, Zuddas, A, editors. *Oxford Textbook of Attention Deficit Hyperactivity Disorder*. Oxford University Press; 2018 May 11.

Kooij, JS. *Adult ADHD: Diagnostic Assessment and treatment*. Springer Science & Business Media; 2012 Dec 11.

Hartman, D, O'Donnell-Killen, T, Doyle, JK, Kavanagh, M, Day, A, Azevedo, J. *The Adult Autism Assessment Handbook: A Neurodiversity Affirmative Approach*. Jessica Kingsley Publishers; 2023 Feb 21.

Hallowell, EM, Ratey, JJ. *ADHD 2.0: New Science and Essential Strategies for Thriving with Distraction – From Childhood Through Adulthood*. Ballantine Books; 2022 Jan 4.

Barkley, RA. *Taking Charge of Adult ADHD: Proven Strategies to Succeed at Work, at Home, and in Relationships*. Guilford Publications; 2021 Sep 14.

Websites:

ADHD UK:
https://adhduk.co.uk/

Young Minds (ADHD and mental health):
https://www.youngminds.org.uk/young-person/mental-health-conditions/adhd-and-mental-health/

ADHD Foundation:
https://www.adhdfoundation.org.uk/resources/

Mind (ADHD and Mental Health):
https://www.mind.org.uk/information-support/tips-for-everyday-living/adhd-and-mental-health/

Attitude:
https://www.additudemag.com/

ADHDADULTUK:
https://www.adhdadult.uk/resources/

National Autistic Society:
https://www.autism.org.uk/

Sensory Direct:
https://www.sensorydirect.com/condition/autism-asd

Beyond Autism:
https://www.beyondautism.org.uk/professionals/services/success-stories/resource-centre/

Bibliography

Abed R, St John-Smith P, editors. *Evolutionary Psychiatry: Current Perspectives on Evolution and Mental Health*. Cambridge University Press; 8 Sep 22.

Antshel KM, Russo N. *Autism Spectrum Disorders and ADHD: Overlapping Phenomenology, Diagnostic Issues, and Treatment Considerations*. Current psychiatry reports. 2019 May;21:1-1.

American Psychiatric Association. *Diagnostic and Statistical Manual of Mental Disorders*.(5th edit) American Psychiatric Association. Washington, DC. 2013.

American Psychiatric Association. *Diagnostic and Statistical Manual of Mental Disorders*.(4th edit) American Psychiatric Association. Washington, DC. 1994.

Bramham J, Ambery F, Young S, Morris R, Russell A, Xenitidis K, Asherson P, Murphy D. "Executive Functioning Differences Between Adults with Attention Deficit Hyperactivity Disorder and Autistic Spectrum Disorder in Initiation, Planning and Strategy Formation". *Autism*. 2009 May;13(3):245-64.

Bush G, Valera EM, Seidman LJ. "Functional Neuroimaging of Attention-deficit/Hyperactivity

Disorder: A Review and Suggested Future Directions". *Biological Psychiatry*. 2005 Jun 1;57(11):1273-84.

Christakou A, Murphy CM, Chantiluke K, Cubillo AI, Smith AB, Giampietro V, Daly E, Ecker C, Robertson D, Murphy DG, Rubia K. "Disorder-specific functional abnormalities during sustained attention in youth with attention deficit hyperactivity disorder (ADHD) and with autism". *Molecular Psychiatry*. 2013 Feb;18(2):236-44.

Matson JL, editor. *Clinical Handbook of ADHD Assessment and Treatment Across the Lifespan*. Springer; 2023 Nov 21.

Davis NO, Kollins SH. "Treatment for Co-occurring Attention Deficit/Hyperactivity Disorder and Autism Spectrum Disorder". *Neurotherapeutics*. 2012 Jul 1;9(3):518-30.

Dupuis A, Mudiyanselage P, Burton CL, Arnold PD, Crosbie J, Schachar RJ. "Hyperfocus or Flow? Attentional Strengths in Autism Spectrum Disorder". *Frontiers in Psychiatry*. 2022 Sep 16;13:886692.

Filipek PA. "Neuroimaging in the Developmental Disorders: The State of the Science". *The Journal of Child Psychology and Psychiatry and Allied Disciplines*. 1999 Jan;40(1):113-28.

Fung LK, editor. *Neurodiversity: From Phenomenology to Neurobiology and Enhancing Technologies*. American Psychiatric Pub; 2021 May 24.

Gargaro BA, Rinehart NJ, Bradshaw JL, Tonge BJ, Sheppard DM. "Autism and ADHD: How Far Have

We Come in the Comorbidity Debate?". *Neuroscience & Biobehavioral Reviews*. 2011 Apr 1;35(5):1081-8.

Goldstein S, Schwebach AJ. "The Comorbidity of Pervasive Developmental Disorder and Attention Deficit Hyperactivity Disorder: Results of a Retrospective Chart Review". *Journal of Autism and Developmental Disorders*. 2004 Jun;34:329-39.

Handen BL, Johnson CR, Lubetsky M. "Efficacy of Methylphenidate Among Children with Autism and Symptoms of Attention-Deficit Hyperactivity Disorder". *Journal of Autism and Developmental Disorders*. 2000 Jun;30:245-55.

Happé F, Booth R, Charlton R, Hughes C. "Executive function deficits in autism spectrum disorders and attention-deficit/hyperactivity disorder: examining profiles across domains and ages". *Brain and Cognition*. 2006 Jun 1;61(1):25-39.

Hazell P. "Drug Therapy for Attention-Deficit/Hyperactivity Disorder-like Symptoms in Autistic Disorder". *Journal of Paediatrics and Child Health*. 2007 Jan;43(1-2):19-24.

Hollander E, Hagerman R, Ferretti C, editors. *Textbook Of Autism Spectrum Disorders*. American Psychiatric Pub; 2022 Mar 15.

Holtmann M, Bölte S, Poustka F. "Attention Deficit Hyperactivity Disorder Symptoms in Pervasive Developmental Disorders: Association with Autistic Behavior Domains and Coexisting Psychopathology". *Psychopathology*. 2007 Feb 22;40(3):172-7.

Hours C, Recasens C, Baleyte JM. "ASD and ADHD Comorbidity: What are we talking about?". *Frontiers in Psychiatry*. 2022 Feb 28;13:837424.

Jang J, Matson JL, Williams LW, Tureck K, Goldin RL, Cervantes PE. "Rates of Comorbid Symptoms in Children with ASD, ADHD, and Comorbid ASD and ADHD". *Research in Developmental Disabilities*. 2013 May 22;34(8):2369-78.

Johnston K, Dittner A, Bramham J, Murphy C, Knight A, Russell A. "Attention Deficit Hyperactivity Disorder Symptoms in Adults with Autism Spectrum Disorders". *Autism Research*. 2013 Aug;6(4):225-36.

Kennedy DM, Banks RS. *The ADHD-Autism Connection: A Step toward More Accurate Diagnoses and Effective Treatments*. Waterbrook Press; 2002.

Kentrou V, de Veld DM, Mataw KJ, Begeer S. "Delayed Autism Spectrum Disorder Recognition in Children and Adolescents Previously Diagnosed with Attention-Deficit/Hyperactivity Disorder". *Autism*. 2019 May;23(4):1065-72.

Kessler RC, Adler L, Ames M, Demler O, Faraone S, Hiripi EV, Howes MJ, Jin R, Secnik K, Spencer T, Ustun TB. "The World Health Organization Adult ADHD Self-Report Scale (ASRS): A Short Screening Scale for Use in the General Population". *Psychological Medicine*. 2005 Feb;35(2):245-56.

Kooij JS. *Adult ADHD: Diagnostic Assessment and Treatment*. Springer Science & Business Media; 2012 Dec 11.

Lai MC, Kassee C, Besney R, Bonato S, Hull L, Mandy W, Szatmari P, Ameis SH. "Prevalence of Co-Occurring Mental Health Diagnoses in the Autism Population: A Systematic Review and Meta-Analysis". *The Lancet Psychiatry*. 2019 Oct 1;6(10):819-29.

Lugo-Marin J, Magan-Maganto M, Rivero-Santana A, Cuellar-Pompa L, Alviani M, Jenaro-Rio C, Diez E, Canal-Bedia R. "Prevalence of Psychiatric Disorders in Adults with Autism Spectrum Disorder: A Systematic Review and Meta-Analysis". *Research in Autism Spectrum Disorders*. 2019 Mar 1;59:22-33.

Lyall K, Schweitzer JB, Schmidt RJ, Hertz-Picciotto I, Solomon M. "Inattention and Hyperactivity in Association with Autism Spectrum Disorders in the CHARGE study". *Research in Autism Spectrum Disorders*. 2017 Mar 1;35:1-2.

Mayes SD, Calhoun SL, Mayes RD, Molitoris S. "Autism and ADHD: Overlapping and Discriminating Symptoms". *Research in Autism Spectrum Disorders*. 2012 Jan 1;6(1):277-85.

Miodovnik A, Harstad E, Sideridis G, Huntington N. "Timing of the Diagnosis of Attention-Deficit/Hyperactivity Disorder and Autism Spectrum Disorder". *Pediatrics*. 2015 Oct 1;136(4):e830-7.

"Attention deficit hyperactivity disorder: diagnosis and management" | Guidance | NICE [Internet]. Nice.org.uk. NICE; 2018. Available from: http://www.nice.org.uk/guidance/NG87.

Nylander L, Holmqvist M, Gustafson L, Gillberg C. "Attention-Deficit/Hyperactivity Disorder (ADHD) and Autism Spectrum Disorder (ASD) in

Adult Psychiatry". A 20-year register study. *Nordic Journal of Psychiatry.* 2013 Oct 1;67(5):344-50.

Banaschewski T, Coghill D, Zuddas A, editors. *Oxford Textbook of Attention Deficit Hyperactivity Disorder.* Oxford University Press; 2018 May 11.

Hollander E, Kolevzon A, Coyle JT. *Textbook of Autism Spectrum Disorders.* Washington, Dc: American Psychiatric Pub; 2011.

Pehlivanidis A, Papanikolaou K, Mantas V, Kalantzi E, Korobili K, Xenaki LA, Vassiliou G, Papageorgiou C. "Lifetime Co-Occurring Psychiatric Disorders in Newly Diagnosed Adults with Attention Deficit Hyperactivity Disorder (ADHD) or/and Autism Spectrum Disorder (ASD)". *BMC Psychiatry.* 2020 Dec;20:1-2.

Price D. *Unmasking Autism: Discovering the New Faces of Neurodiversity.* Harmony; 2022 Apr 5.

Rao PA, Landa RJ. "Association Between Severity of Behavioral Phenotype and Comorbid Attention Deficit Hyperactivity Disorder Symptoms in Children with Autism Spectrum Disorders". *Autism.* 2014 Apr;18(3):272-80.

Rommelse N, Buitelaar JK, Hartman CA. "Structural Brain Imaging Correlates of ASD and ADHD Across the Lifespan: A Hypothesis-Generating Review on Developmental ASD–ADHD Subtypes". *Journal of Neural Transmission.* 2017 Feb;124:259-71.

Rong Y, Yang CJ, Jin Y, Wang Y. "Prevalence of Attention-Deficit/Hyperactivity Disorder in Individuals with Autism Spectrum Disorder:

A Meta-Analysis". *Research in Autism Spectrum Disorders.* 2021 May 1;83:101759.

Simonoff E, Pickles A, Charman T, Chandler S, Loucas T, Baird G. "Psychiatric Disorders in Children with Autism Spectrum Disorders: Prevalence, Comorbidity, and Associated Factors in a Population-Derived Sample". *Journal of the American Academy of Child & Adolescent Psychiatry.* 2008 Aug 1;47(8):921-9.

Stahl SM, Mignon L. *Stahl's Illustrated Attention Deficit Hyperactivity Disorder.* Cambridge University Press; 2009 Aug 24.

Stevens T, Peng L, Barnard-Brak L. "The Comorbidity of ADHD in Children Diagnosed with Autism Spectrum Disorder". *Research in Autism Spectrum Disorders.* 2016 Nov 1;31:11-8.

Sysoeva OV. "Neurophysiological Markers that Link Genes and Behavior in Humans: Examples from Rare Genetic Syndromes Associated with Autism Spectrum Disorders". *Genes & Cells.* 2023 Dec 15;18(4):297-307.

Taylor MJ, Charman T, Robinson EB, Plomin R, Happé F, Asherson P, Ronald A. "Developmental Associations Between Traits of Autism Spectrum Disorder and Attention Deficit Hyperactivity Disorder: A Genetically Informative, Longitudinal Twin Study". *Psychological Medicine.* 2013 Aug;43(8):1735-46.

Taylor E. "Development of the Concept". *Oxford Textbook of Attention Deficit Hyperactivity Disorder.* Oxford University Press, Oxford. 2018 May 24.

White SW, Maddox BB, Mazefsky CA, editors. *The Oxford Handbook of Autism And Co-Occurring Psychiatric Conditions*. Oxford University Press; 2020 Feb 3.

van Steijn DJ, Richards JS, Oerlemans AM, de Ruiter SW, van Aken MA, Franke B, Buitelaar JK, Rommelse NN. "The co-occurrence of autism spectrum disorder and attention-deficit/hyperactivity disorder symptoms in parents of children with ASD or ASD with ADHD". *Journal of Child Psychology and Psychiatry*. 2012 Sep;53(9):954-63.

World Health Organization. *International Classification of Diseases for Mortality and Morbidity Statistics* (11th Revision) [Internet]. 2018 Feb 4.

Witwer AN, Lecavalier L. "Validity of Comorbid Psychiatric Disorders in Youngsters with Autism Spectrum Disorders". *Journal of Developmental and Physical Disabilities*. 2010 Aug;22:367-80.

Yang J, Zhou SJ, Zhang LY, Ding Y, Zhang G. "The relationship between theory of mind and executive function: Evidence from children with ASD or ADHD". *Chinese Journal of Clinical Psychology*. 2008 Jun.

Zachor DA, Ben-Itzchak E. "From toddlerhood to adolescence, trajectories and predictors of outcome: Long-term follow-up study in autism spectrum disorder". *Autism Research*. 2020 Jul;13(7):1130-43.